Theatre Routine

MODERN PRACTICAL NURSING SERIES

This important new nursing series, designed specifically for the State Enrolled Nurse and Auxilliary Nurse is published as a 'parent' book covering the basic nursing skills entitled AN OUTLINE OF BASIC NURSING CARE, and a number of smaller handbooks covering the individual specialities as the nurse is moved from one discipline to another.

AN OUTLINE OF BASIC NURSING CARE: This aims to help the nurse learn the general basic nursing skills and also how to apply them, and to stimulate thought about nursing in differing hospital situations.

THE SPECIALITY BOOKS: Having mastered the basic nursing skills the pupil nurse will find herself attached to the nursing staff in any ward in the hospital. Although she is expected to play a part in this specialised ward team she may have had only a brief glimpse of the subject in her earlier training. It is for this stage in her career that this series of books is designed. The subjects covered include: Paediatric Orthopaedics, Theatre Routine, Paediatric Surgery, Dermatology, Urology, Adult Medicine, Geriatrics, Ear Nose and Throat, Mental Deficiency, Ophthalmology, Adult Orthopaedics, Plastics and Burns, Psychiatry, Obstetrics and Adult Surgery. All these are written by expert authors usually consisting of a doctor and sister tutor actively engaged in the work about which they have written and in touch with modern nursing trends.

These books are extensively illustrated and easy to use. As paperbacks they are inexpensive and it is hoped therefore that the nurse will have available a set of modern practical books which will help her in her ward work.

2 Modern Practical Nursing Series

Theatre Routine

Morag H. Campbell, R.G.N., S.C.M.
Senior Nursing Officer (Theatres & C.S.S.D.)
Royal Infirmary Glasgow

WILLIAM HEINEMANN MEDICAL BOOKS LIMITED:
LONDON

This book is dedicated to you.
I hope you enjoy working in Theatre as much as I do.

First published 1971

ISBN 0 433 05138 8

Printed in Great Britain by
The Redwood Press Ltd., Trowbridge.

Contents

Preface

This book is designed to answer the thousand and one questions an intelligent nurse would ask when she first started to work in an operating theatre.

The book has been presented in that form.

The nurse must however realise that although broadly speaking techniques do not alter in the ends they achieve there are considerable local variations in their application.

It is therefore one of her first duties to find out how things are done in the particular operating suite she finds herself working .

There are a few blank pages in this book and it is wise to use them to note any particular points you may learn as you go along.

Some day you may be the senior nurse and then–by referring to your own notes–realise what you can tell the newcomer.

M. C.

1 Operating Theatre Nursing

The patient needs the nurse to care for him in the operating theatre just as he does in the hospital ward.

Theatre nursing is a special branch of nursing just as the surgeon and the anaesthetist are members of special branches of the medical profession. The theatre nurse is also a member of a team of many, all working to provide a safe passage through the operating theatre for every patient.

Off-duty interests play a big part in making the theatre nurse a vital member of the team. She will benefit from having lots of fresh air, regular meals, and active participation in other activities.

However small or insignificant the task to be performed the theatre nurse feels responsible in some small way for the success of the procedure.

In the operating theatre expert nurses–highly skilled and trained–are needed for the patient's benefit at a very important stage in his hospital stay.

What are the qualities required in a Theatre Nurse?

1 A placid nature with qualities of kindness and patience.
2 A real desire to be a theatre nurse.
3 A sense of responsibility.
4 The ability to co-operate with all members of the team.
5 Good powers of observation and a bright enquiring mind.
6 A vital, interested, and enthusiastic disposition.
7 The ability to accept changes.
8 A healthy and proud appearance.

9 A bright attitude to life in general.

What are the aims of a Theatre Nurse?

1 To allay the fears of the patient.
2 To integrate the patient care during his period in theatre.
3 To become expert and highly skilled in the theatre techniques.
4 To develop speed and accuracy in these techniques.
5 To be able to impart knowledge to others.
6 To prepare conscientiously by study for the changing world of medicine.

What does the Surgeon expect of the Theatre Nurse?

PERFECTION!

2

Why are Operations Performed in an Operating Theatre?

Operating theatres are found in many different situations.

Sometimes a single Theatre Suite is situated beside a ward or a group of wards and solely used by the patients and staff from that group of wards.

Twin Theatre Suites are fairly common perhaps serving one or two different surgical specialties.

A central Theatre Suite is more common in the new hospital complexes. In the modern planning of theatre suites many more theatres (4-8 theatres) are incorporated in one large area.

In this case many of the facilities and rooms are shared by all of the staff. The surgeons here operate on a sessional basis e.g. perhaps in the morning an Ear, Nose, and Throat surgeon may be operating and in the afternoon a General surgeon may operate.

To the outside world the word 'theatre' is the place where the production of some stage show or play is performed by a group of actors. It might also be the place where a new concerto is played by an orchestra of musicians. An operating theatre is very much likened to this. It is set for the tuning up of an efficient team of staff and instruments for the performance of an operation or operations.

Rehearsals may take place to give a perfect musical performance. Theatre staff too are rehearsed and trained to give perfect operation team performance.

A good team can be likened to a corps de ballet. No word need be spoken. Each member of the team can anticipate the other's needs and actions.

An operating theatre should have a bacterial free enviroment.

There is a place for everything and everything is in its place.

The atmosphere must be a happy one and as free from tension as is possible in the circumstances.

Operations are performed there because all the trained personnel are there. It is a highly specialised branch of nursing.

3
Where are the Various Rooms in the Operating Theatre?

Reception Room or Area

This is the room where the staff–including the nurse–receives the patient into the operating area.

The patient may be removed from the trolley to the operating table in this area, perhaps he may be anaesthetised on his trolley and then transferred to the operating table.

To prevent cross-infection great care is taken to substitute clean theatre clothing and blankets before entering the theatre area.

Anaesthetic Room

This is the room where the patient receives the anaesthetic in quietness. Correct positioning for the particular operation is carried out here. This procedure however varies a great deal according to local hospital preferences.

Operating Theatre

The patient is taken here usually after the induction of anaesthesia. The theatre is prepared beforehand and the equipment is all in place for the particular type of operation expected.

All personnel within the theatre are ready to perform their respective duties.

Preparation or Laying-up Room

This varies according to the plan of the operating room or suite. Packets, instruments, trays, and other materials sterilised for use are stored in this room ready to be used in the operating theatre.

Trolleys are stocked here with all the requirements anticipated for the operation which will follow.

If pre-set instruments are not used then the trolley may be completely laid in this room. Obviously it must be situated adjacent to the theatre.

Sluice or Disposal Room

All used trolleys and materials from the theatre are placed in this room. These articles are cleaned and made ready for re-sterilisation or are disposed of in appropriate containers.

In some modern theatre suites this used material is taken straight to a central department and processed there e.g. Theatre Sterile Service Unit.

Scrub-up Room or Bay

This may be an alcove or a separate room where personnel to be scrubbed for the operation prepare their hands and arms. If there is adequate room the procedure of donning gowns and gloves may take place here also.

Sterile Store

All sterile articles are stored in this room ready to be transferred when required in the laying-up area.

Unsterile Store or Packing Area

This may not be available as a separate room. Here articles awaiting packing prior to sterilisation are kept. e.g. all dressings, materials, instruments, linen, drains, and other sundry stocks.

Equipment Store

This also may not always be available but it is very useful for the storage of all machinery, parts of the table rarely used, furniture etc.

Plaster Room

This room may be part of a theatre suite where orthopaedic surgery is carried out.

Changing Room

These are available for male and female staff. Toilet and shower facilities are usually available. These rooms are usually arranged so that staff can change clothing and footwear before entering the clean area.

Barrier Area

This may or may not be present. Sometimes there is a clean corridor between changing areas and theatres. At some point footwear is changed. There are many variations of interchange areas.

Recovery Area

This explains itself. Ideally patients are kept in this area for up to an hour after operation until consciousness is fully restored.

4 What is Worn in the Operating Theatre?

Special clothing is worn before entering the operating theatre for each operating session. This clothing may be changed also after an operation where the wound is infected.

In some theatre suites it may be the rule for personnel to have a shower prior to changing into theatre clothing.

All staff working in theatre must also be aware of any septic leison on their skin or any source of infection and report this immediately to their appropriate head of department. This infection must be cleared before return to duty.

Dress or Trouser Suit

This should be well-fitting, freshly laundered, and attractive.

It is usually without pockets. If a belt is attached this should not be tied at the front of the dress or suit, thus preventing any contamination when coming into contact with sterile trolleys etc.

Grades of staff may be identified by different colours of theatre dress or other methods of distinction.

Sleeves are kept fairly short so that elbow areas are free for scrubbing.

Caps

The styles of these vary a great deal. Disposable caps are available. The important point to remember is that all the hair is completely covered. Each person develops his or her own preference of style according to hair style. Hair must be kept as neat, clean and tidy as possible.

Stockings or Socks

This is also a matter of preference but of course must be frequently washed.

Shoes

It is important that footwear is comfortable and easily cleaned. They should also be anti-static. Quite frequently clogs are worn. These are very comfortable when long periods of standing are involved.

Sandshoes tend to make the feet hot and sticky and tired.

Sandals tend to be noisy and cause slipping.

All footwear must be washed after each period of use.

Masks

There are many varieties of masks. Disposable and otherwise are available in great abundance. Masks should be changed frequently and never re-applied when pulled from the face. A mask is removed by the tapes to prevent contamination of the hands. It is discarded immediately after use and the hands are washed.

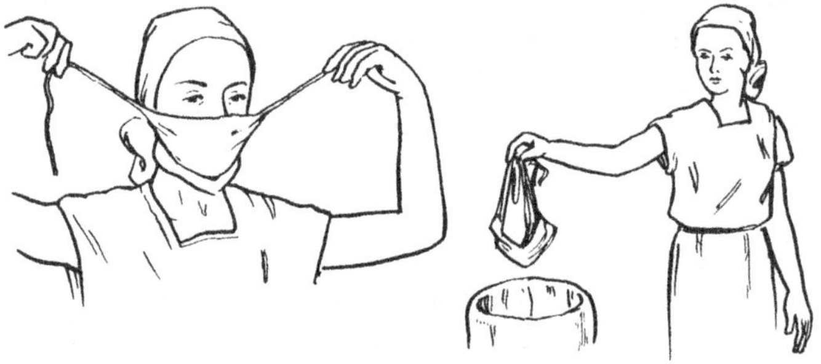

Fig. 1

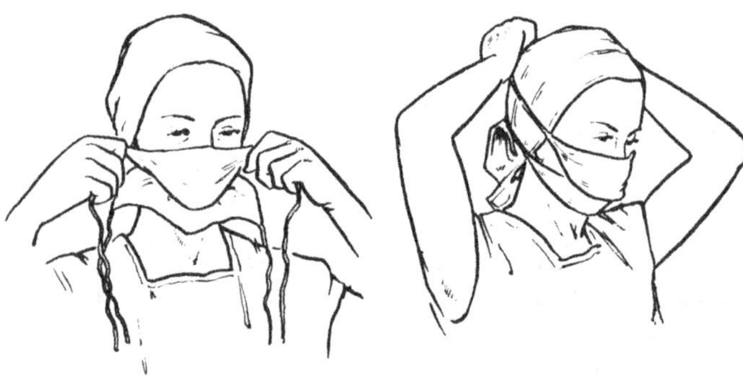

Fig. 2

Jewellery

It is preferable that this is not worn. It is liable to cause injury to the patient or to be damaged itself. Wedding rings are a source of controversy both from the infection and the static electricity point of view.

Make-up and General Appearance

Cosmetics can be applied in moderation. Nail varnish should not be worn. The patient will be reassured if the theatre nurse presents a neat, composed, professional appearance.

5
What is the Basic Furniture in the Operating Theatre?

Basin Stand

This is a basin holder on wheels. It is placed by the circulating nurse in a suitable spot in the theatre convenient to the surgeon or 'scrub' nurse. A basin (polypropylene or stainless steel) is sterilised inside suitable wrappings and put in the stand.

It is opened out as the operation commences and sterile water or other lotion may be added by the circulating nurse.

Trolleys

There are many varieties of trolley. The number of them, the shape of those used, and the position during operation depend on the type of surgery carried out in that particular theatre. The trolley itself should not have sides. This prevents the risk of contamination.

The top shelf in modern trolleys is flush with the corners to aid cleaning.

The trolley may have one or two shelves.

Mayo Table

This is an aid to the instrument nurse. It can be on wheels or as a fitment to the operating table. Always the height of the Mayo table is adjustable. Care must be taken that it never rests on the patient's limbs and that this point is checked if the position of the patient is changed.

Run-about Buckets

These are small bins on wheels. They are placed usually on the right hand of both the surgeon and the assistants. One is also made available for the instrument nurse. A paper lining can be used in these bins to prevent any handling of dirty material between operations.

Diathermy Apparatus

This can be a portable machine fitted to the base of an operating table, or fitted to an overhead boom, or fitted (into a suitable socket) in the operating theatre wall.

A foot pedal is part of this apparatus. This is placed in a suitable position for the surgeon. The diathermy apparatus is used to cauterise bleeding vessels.

Suction Apparatus

This can be operated from a central suction unit or be an individual portable suction apparatus. There are normally two sets of suction available—one for the needs of of the anaesthetist and one for the needs of the surgeon.

Operating Table

This varies according to the type of surgery performed. In the main the operating table is moveable, the patient being transferred from a trolley to the table either outside the operating theatre itself or occasionally in the theatre. One type of table has various trolley tops. The trolley top is placed on a permanent base fixed in position in the operating theatre.

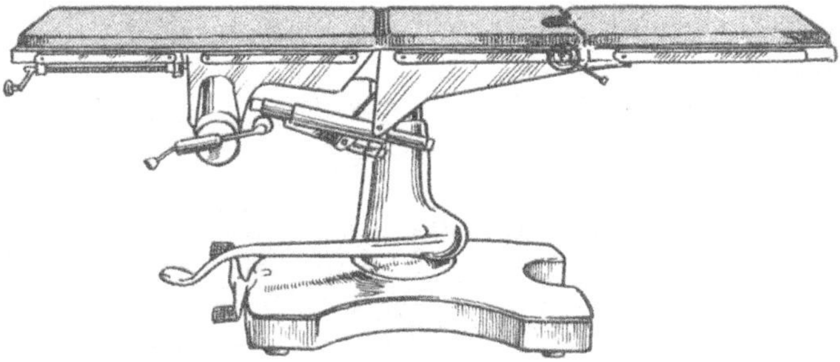

Fig. 3 Operating Table

Anaesthetic Machine

Usually one machine or apparatus remains in the theatre and the patient is connected up to this on entry to the operating theatre. The gases may be lead from a piped gas supply or from cylinders of the gases attached to the machine. Suction may also be part of the machine.

Drip Stand

This of course is usually mobile and may be fitted with a pump for quick transfusion.

Operating Lights

These may be fixtures to the ceiling. For instance one satelite light attached to the large centre light.

Alternatively the surgeon may prefer two or more portable lights.

Viewing Screens

These screens are almost always fitted flush to the walls. They may or may not be fitted with drip trays for use with wet plates.

Swab Rack

This is present in all theatres. It can be a simple rod detachable for cleaning or a large board of stainless steel with three or more rows of hooks or holes in multiples of ten. This enables the circulating nurse to hang up swabs during the operation.

These pieces of furniture mentioned are only a few of the main pieces of operating theatre furniture.

6

How is the Theatre and the Theatre Equipment Cleaned Prior to Operation?

Specific routine cleaning procedures are scheduled at regular time intervals to ensure that all apparatus, equipment, and areas have the correct cleaning and maintainance. Some of these procedures will be carried out by the operating theatre staff; others by cleaning teams; and some by painters, engineers, and maintainance staff. The important point is that those programmes are adhered to and that all staff are trained to carry them out.

A High Standard of Cleanliness is Essential

Walls

These are washed in most instances once per day. In new theatre suites automatic spraying can be employed, provided electrical points are fitted with waterproof covers and that other apparatus can be protected.

Furniture

The same strength of antiseptic is used to wash all theatre furniture. Conscientiousness is important. Furniture is cleaned thoroughly and in strict rotation around the theatre. Detachable parts of any piece of furniture are first removed and washed separately. e.g. If a trolley has detachable shelves these are removed, washed, and placed on a clean surface. The base is then washed and the clean shelves are replaced in position. Particular attention is paid to the wheels of furniture as dirt and suture threads quickly gather making the article less mobile. It is essential that furniture moves freely and smoothly at all times.

Lights

The operating lights can sometimes be missed. They are washed by the same method. A special fluid can be used on the glass to prevent smudging.

Floors

The floor can be cleaned by an operator using a scrubbing

machine preferably after each operation session. Usually a sponge mop immersed in the antiseptic lotion is used to clean the floor between operations.

Suction Apparatus

A solution of mild antiseptic is allowed to be sucked through the tubing. If the tubing is disposable then it is discarded. If it is not disposable then the tubing is removed for further cleaning before re-sterilisation. The bottles are emptied, cleaned and re-sterilised. If the contents of the bottles are infected then antiseptic is added. After the necessary period of soaking the fluid is discarded and the cleaning and sterilisation process takes place.

Operating Table

The mattress is removed, washed, dried, and placed on a clean surface. The actual table is thoroughly washed paying particular attention to all joints. It is dried before the mattress is replaced. The base of the table is very often forgotten about and has been found to be a source of infection. This should be cleaned at regular intervals but suitable trained help must be available to tilt the table properly for this procedure.

Accessories for the Table

The pillows and all table fitments are cleaned thoroughly, dried, and replaced either on to the table or in readiness for further use.

If any wet rubber comes into contact with the metal parts of the table it will cause staining of the table or fitments, as antistatic rubber readily adheres when it is wet.

Diathermy Apparatus

This is washed with other theatre furniture. The foot piece is sometimes difficult to clean. It should not be soaked as this will cause damage to it. The apparatus is checked after washing. All dials are turned to zero and the machine is made ready for use again.

Anaesthetic Machine

This is washed in the same way. All apparatus used at the previous operation is removed. If suction apparatus is fitted to the machine this is cleaned as previously described (page 14). The machine is checked and clean routine equipment is laid ready. The corrugated tubing can be treated either by soaking in an antiseptic for a stated period or sterilising in a 'flash' autoclave if one is available. The latter method should not be routine but can be used for tubing that has been used on a patient with a known infection e.g. T.B.

The theatre nurse should be familiar with the method of cleaning each piece of equipment and each instrument. It is not always her duty to do the actual cleaning but she must be able to advise and supervise this important part of theatre work.

7

How is a Theatre Prepared for Operation?

The preparation of theatre involves the whole operating team and each member has a specific duty to perform.

The Daily Cleaning Schedule

This is carried out under the direct supervision of the nursing staff in the operating theatre. The nursing staff must be trained in this.

The Furniture and Equipment

Furniture in the actual operating theatre is then placed in the correct position for the particular operation on the operating list.

Pieces of equipment additional to the basic are also put in place if required e.g. an arm table for an operation on the hand or arm,

Equipment

All equipment must be checked to be in good working order. This will include the operating lights and the diathermy machine. The foot plate is placed out in the required position for the surgeon's use and the dials are at the appropriate setting. In particular all suction apparatus is checked to be complete with tubing, the catheter attached, and tested for efficiency.

Pre-sterilised Basic Packs, Instrument Trays, and Supplementary Packs

These are collected from the sterile store by trolley. Information from the operating list will be required. The surgeon and assistants stated on the list will determine the gloves ready for use, the suture material required, and any other specialities particular to the surgeon.

The packs are taken to the operating theatre and each pack is placed in the position from which it will be opened in due course.

Operation Cards or Books

These cards or books are available in most operating theatres. They are compiled with all information of the requirements for a particular operation and by a particular surgeon. As the nurse gains experience, her anticipation of requirements for each operation will steadily become more perfect. It is essential that the information on the cards is kept up to date as changes occur.

Sterile Basins or Bowls

These are put into basin stands ready to be opened out.

Sterile Nail Brush Dispensers and Gown Packs

These are laid out in the scrubbing-up area.

Special Drugs, Lotions, and Sterile Water

These should always be available in adequate quantity.

Temperature and Humidity

The temperature and humidity of the operating theatre are checked. The temperature is routinely 20°-22°C. (68°-72°F.). It may have to be raised or lowered for particular operations or particular patients e.g. it will be raised if a baby is requiring an operation.

The humidity in the operating theatre should be 50-55%.

Special Apparatus

When required special apparatus is made ready e.g. an orthopaedic table or equipment for cholangiogram.

The Swab Chart or Board

This is prepared in readiness for the count of swabs following surgery.

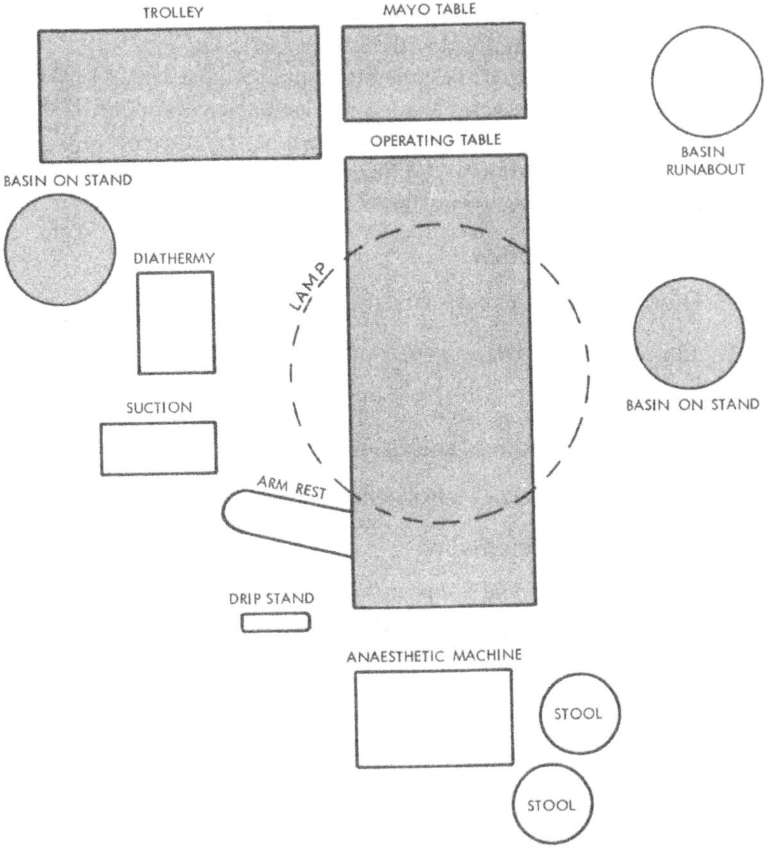

Fig. 4

Plan showing position of basic requirements for an Operating Theatre

Anaesthetic Room

Again the furniture, table, anaesthetic machine, and other equipment are positioned in readiness. A standard procedure of laying out equipment and drugs is carried out. It is important that the anaesthetist can check all his requirements quickly and have ease of access to these. The anaesthetic machine is checked by the attendant or anaesthetic nurse but is always rechecked by the anaesthetist. A check of cylinders is important if piped gases are not available. In this room the patient is usually put in position for the operation therefore all the table accessories for the required position should be in readiness before the patient arrives.

The diathermy electrode is available for attachment to the patient along with the contact cream or isotonic saline.

Intravenous fluid infusion apparatus should be prepared. Knowledge of blood availability should be known by the staff assisting in the anaesthetic room. A well prepared list will also help the staff in the anaesthetic room to have all the required equipment available e.g. for a local anaesthetic, or a spinal anaesthetic.

Sometimes an actual procedure will be carried out prior to the patient going into the operating theatre e.g. a bronchoscopy.

A well-prepared theatre means a smooth-running operation.

8

How are Articles Packed for Sterilisation?

The preparation of packs is not always the duty of the

theatre nurse but it is important that she is aware of the principles involved.

There are two main types of packs that can be prepared in the theatre area.

1 Large Basic Pack of Drapes and Swabs to be opened out on to a Trolley

There are two wraps required. These can be made of double thickness closely woven cotton or of wrapping paper suitable for this purpose which will permit steam penetration.

Two colours of wrap or two different materials e.g. outer paper and inner cotton may be the routine. This enables the nurse to identify each stage of the opening of the pack more easily.

The wrap must be large enough to drape over the sides of the trolley that is used in theatre (approximately 54" or 137cm. square). Both wraps are placed together on the packing table.

The contents in the order in which they are going to be used are positioned in the middle of the wraps. Taking the inner wrap lengthwise it is brought over the contents and the extra piece brought back as a flap or cuff. This is repeated with the opposite flap. The sides are then brought up to come over the pack again. The pack is now secured with a piece of autoclave tape. This procedure is repeated again using the outer wrap and again secured with autoclave tape. The pack may or may not be placed in a paper bag forming a dust cover. Alternatively the packet can be placed in a transparent dust cover bag after sterilisation. This packet is now labelled with the contents, the date of sterilisation, and sometimes the initials of the packer.

2 Envelope Packet

Again two wraps which are square are required. The article

or articles to be wrapped are placed diagonally in the centre of the inner square. The corner is brought over the contents and the tip folded back to form a cuff. The two side pieces are folded to the centre in the same way. The farthest away corner is now folded on top of the others. This packet is then placed in the outer square and wrapped by the same method. The last corner is secured with autoclave tape and labelling carried out as before.

These two methods can be used for packing most articles.

Articles not Packed in the Operating Theatre

These will almost certainly be prepared in the Central Sterile Supply Department. Included in this will be instruments perhaps for dry heat sterilisation. These will be placed in aluminium tins sealed with foil caps.

The Pre-set Trays

These trays will be packed in the Theatre Sterile Service Unit. There are two ways of preparing the instruments and drapes for an operation in a central department:-

1 One single pack containing a basic instrument set placed in order on a tray. On top of the instruments are positioned the dressings and towels in correct order of use. When placing the tray on the outer and inner wraps care should be taken that the tray will be in the correct position when it is opened on the trolley i.e. more to the one end of the pack cover.
2 Two packets are prepared. One will have the instruments in order on a tray, the other will contain the dressings and drapes.

The pack well-prepared before sterilisation makes for a more efficient and safe presentation at the operating table after sterilisation.

9
What are the Various Methods of Sterilisation?

What is Sterile?

An article is sterile after being through a sterilising process. This means it has been cleaned, packed, labelled, dated, sterilised, and stored until it is required for use at the operation site.

This sterilising process may take place outside the hospital in a Central Sterile Supply Department, in a hospital, or maybe in the theatre area.

The important fact to remember is that there is only one way to carry out this sterilisation process and that is the correct way. There is no such state as 'nearly sterile' or 'almost sterile'.

Equipment is *sterile* or it is *not sterile.*

Sterilisation is the Complete Destruction of all Living Microbes

Any discrepancy regarding packaging, date, or identification should be reported immediately. Some articles cannot be sterilised and can only be disinfected. Equipment for sterilisation varies in each hospital and theatre area. Some hospitals have a Central Sterile Department, others have to carry out many sterilisation methods in the theatre area. Here are a few methods described as simply as possible.

The Agents of Sterilisation

1 moist heat
2 dry heat

3 chemicals
4 gas or vapour
5 irradiation

1 Moist Heat (Steam under Pressure)

This type of sterilising is carried out using an autoclave. It is considered to be the safest and most practical means of sterilising linen, materials, fluids, and the majority of instruments. Steam under pressure permits penetration of moist heat to porous substances and results in the destruction of all microbes.

A close-fitting vessel is necessary to attain steam under pressure e.g. a pressure cooker.

The higher the steam pressure, the higher the temperature becomes. The steam is the sterilising agent. If steam is mixed with air the temperature will be lower. The air acts as a barrier to steam penetration. In hospital we use an *autoclave* as the close-fitting vessel.

The Autoclave

The machine consists of two metal cylinders—one within the other. Between the cylinders is an enclosed space known as the jacket in which steam and heat can be maintained at a considerably high pressure. The autoclave is fitted with various gauges, valves, thermometers, etc. There are certain steps in the autoclaving of any article.

Loading Process

1 Packaging and wrapping of articles and then of loading them into the steriliser are important factors which govern the effectiveness of steam sterilisation.
2 Fabrics must be freshly laundered in order to enable the steam to penetrate the fibres sufficiently.
3 Pack covers must protect the material or article to be

sterilised from contamination and must also serve as effective dust filters. They must also pass a thickness and permeability test as must paper if it used as a wrap. Cotton is considered to be a good material for a pack cover.

4 The dating of the pack makes sure that storage is not too prolonged. Shelf life exposes goods to the hazards of dust, frequent handling, and accidental contamination. Expiry dates vary with different conditions.

5 The chamber is loaded in such a way that there is little resistance to the passage of steam.

6 Packs should be placed in the autoclave on edge or in a vertical position.

Sterilising Process

When the doors and valves of the autoclave are closed the pressure inside rises with a resulting increase in the steam temperature.

It is essential to have air evacuated in order to permit the proper penetration of steam. The steam forces the air out completely in an effective autoclave. This will then give a full sterilisation temperature. This temperature is held for a fixed period e.g. 134°C or 274°F for three minutes.

After this sterilising period a vacuum is drawn removing the steam and replacing it with filtered air.

When packets are removed from the autoclave they should not be stacked one on top of the other. Air must be allowed to circulate around.

They should never be put on a metal surface or rapid condensation will cause the packets to become wet and liable to the risk of contamination.

Packets should be stored in clean ventilated conditions.

Autoclave Tests on High Pressure High Vacuum Autoclaves

These are many and varied and are carried out by personnel in the hospital.

Indicator tapes are familiar to the theatre nursing staff. The tapes used show only that they have been exposed to steam for a period of time at a temperature sufficient to affect them. This brings about the colour change on the markings. There are various forms of tape. The most common is the 3M. Autoclave Tape where the cross markings become uniformly brown after being exposed to this steam.

Bowie-Dick Test

This is an important and practical method of testing an autoclave's efficiency. Sterilising attendants can carry out this test. A test pack consists of freshly laundered huckaback towels. Each towel is folded into eight thicknesses and made to form a stack measuring ten to eleven inches. (250cm).

A piece of paper to which autoclave tape has been applied in the form of a cross diagonally is placed on the middle of the pack. It is important that this pack is placed in the centre of the autoclave by itself. If all the air is not removed it will be forced into the centre of the pack and consequently the temperature will be lowered and the tape will not change in the centre of the cross in the same degree as the edges.

Other tests include Leak Tests, Culture Tests, and the use of temperature recording apparatus.

In the theatre area autoclaves with no post-vacuum are sometimes found. This type is very often used for the "dropped" instrument. It is a quick method of sterilising instruments for immediate use. There is no drying period and therefore no article can be wrapped and sterilised in this autoclave.

Boiling

Contrary to popular and past belief boiling does not sterilise. Resistant spores can survive boiling temperatures.

Fluid Sterilizing Autoclave

This is similar in sterilising process to the autoclave already described (page 23). Pressure in the steriliser must be exhausted slowly. A rapid cooling device is also fitted. Sterile water for use in theatre is sterilised by this method. The bottles are fitted with a vacuum cap.

Infusion fluids and pharmacy solutions are also prepared by this method.

2 Dry Heat—Hot Air Oven

This method is used for materials like glass, powder and oils. It is also suitable for sterilising instruments with inner greased parts e.g. an automatic bone saw or drill. It is also sometimes used for sterilising very fine instruments.

The temperature is held at 160°C for a period of one hour but this may vary with the packaging, wrapping, and material to be sterilised.

Hot Air Oven Test

For this test 3M Tape (Hot Air Tape) or Browne's tubes with a green spot can be used. The tape changes to a pink colour after the correct temperature has been held in the oven. The tube changes from red to green.

Infra-Red Radiation

Infra-Red Radiation is another dry heat method of sterilisation. This heat is very often conducted on to a conveyor belt. Ward instruments are sometimes sterilised in this way in C.S.S.D. departments.

3 Chemicals

There is a great variety of chemicals available. It is important that the nurse knows in a particular operating theatre the specific chemical that is used to destroy spores and sterilise the article in question.

Only articles or instruments that cannot be sterilised by any other method should be subjected to chemical sterilisation. The instruments most commonly treated by this method are those with lenses e.g. cystoscopes.

The User of Chemicals must know the following Facts

1. The strength of the chemical. A suitable measure to obtain this strength is required.
2. The length of time required for the chemical is to kill spores.
3. Why it is necessary to use this method of sterilisation.
4. Which microbes are affected by the particular chemical.

4 Gas and Vapour

Ethylene Oxide

There are varying opinions as to the efficiency of this method of sterilisation. It is used to sterilise heat-sensitive materials like plastics and many articles previously sterilised in chemicals.

The cycle of an ethylene oxide steriliser is quite similar to that of an autoclave with pre-vacuum, sterilising, and post-vacuum periods. It is essential that all articles are thoroughly cleaned, dried, and carefully inspected before packing. Low density polythene film is used for packing the articles.

As much air as possible is extracted from the packs and they are sealed with a heat-sealing machine. All packaging must be done in a room with a high atmospheric humidity (50% or more).

After the sterilising process it is necessary to 'air' the processed articles in order to remove all the gas retained in the packaging. The time limit is over twelve hours for most articles.

Ethylene Oxide Test

For this test 3M Ethylene Oxide Tape is used. The background (green) changes colour, instead of the stripes across the tape, as in the other tapes.

Low Pressure Steam with Formaldehyde

This is the exposure to steam at sub-atmospheric pressure with the addition of a prescribed measured quantity of formaldehyde. This is not generally in use.

Formaldehyde Vapour

Tablets provide this vapour. It does not penetrate well but may be used for endoscopic instruments. The time involved is very long (approximately twelve hours).

5 Irradiation

The most usual technique is to use gamma rays from radio-active sources e.g. Cobalt 60. Good penetration can be obtained and closed packs can be processed. There is no residual radio-activity. This form of sterilisation is carried out at a few centres in Great Britain on an industrial basis. It is commonly used by industry for many disposable articles supplied to hospitals.

A knowledge of the method of sterilising each article used in the operating theatre is essential to the nurse even though it may not be her duty to carry out the sterilising process.

10

What are the Antistatic Precautions in the Operating Theatre?

Static electricity is a hazard in the operating theatre so long as inflammable gases such as cyclopropane and ether are used as anaesthetics.

Basically no materials that generate electricity should be allowed into the operating theatre. All movable furniture and equipment should be electrically connected via the floor—that is—have anti-static wheels.

All personnel should wear anti-static footwear.

Any rubber sheeting used in table fitments, covers, and pillows should be of the anti-static variety. This anti-static material must be regularly tested by the maintainance department for conductivity.

The colours black, or black and yellow immediately identify the material.

Points to Note

1 Woollen blankets and many man-made fibres are most dangerous and should not be allowed in the operating theatre.

2 Cotton is a most suitable material and the over-garments of the theatre personnel should be made of this.
3 Apparatus and materials stored in plastic covers should not be stored in the theatre area. Static electricity can build up if there is friction of one surface on another.
4 Diathermy and X-ray equipment must never be used if an inflammable gas is present in the operating theatre.
5 Skin cleaning materials containing spirit are to be discouraged.
6 Aerosol sprays are also a source of danger and should be carefully used.
7 Electrical equipment must be tested to be explosive-proof before being introduced to the operating area. All such apparatus in Great Britain must by regulation be 4' 6" (137cm.) above floor level.
8 Electric switches must be explosive-proof on installation.
9 A regular inspection and maintainance programme is essential.
10 A special store for the inflammable gases should be positioned well away from the high risk area.
11 Humidity in the theatre should be maintained at 50%-55%.

Theatre personnel must be constantly aware of the dangers of static electricity.

11
How is the Patient Received and Cared for in the Operating Theatre?

Each Patient is a Life

This life must be protected by safety measures.

We take care of our own lives when we are crossing a road etc. so we must also take care of the patient who entrusts his life with us when he comes to the operating theatre.

We must remember that he will be unconscious and not able to feel sensation. Consequently he will not be able to tell us of any pain he may feel.

He is unable to complain of any physical discomfort which he would not normally tolerate.

Everyone who comes into hospital for an operation has fears—no matter how trivial the operation may be.

Where it is practical the theatre nurse can help the patients allay these fears by visiting them in the ward the evening before surgery. The patient will appreciate the fact that he knows someone in the theatre.

Most people have no idea of the methods of 'going to sleep' and the theatre nurse can explain this and perhaps be able to inspire the patient's confidence.

On Arrival at the Theatre

It is important that the patient is greeted pleasantly by his name. This re-assures him that he is recognised as an individual. He must not be made to feel that he is part of an 'assembly line' but that the staff will care for him personally and particularly during this critical period of his hospital stay.

Even though the nurse greeting him may well be wearing a mask her eyes can still reflect a pleasant expression.

The manner in which a nurse moves about her work can also have an effect on the patient.

Brief explanations to the patient of the procedures being carried out by the nursing and medical staff are essential e.g. the blankets may be changed, a tourniquet may be applied, or an injection may be about to be given by the anaesthetist.

Each patient should be assessed individually. One patient may want to chat, another will want to be listened to, and yet another will want to be talked to and re-assured.

Transference of Patients

The transfer of patients depends on the transfer or barrier area at the entrance to the theatre, and also whether the patient comes to theatre in his own bed or on a trolley.

The routine will vary between different theatre areas. Transfer can take place between bed and operating table, trolley and operating table, and ward trolley and theatre trolley.

The patient may be lifted by the staff manually or on a stretcher.

Precautions to Take

It is most important to observe certain precautions whichever method is used.

1 The vehicle must be held securely. The wheel locking devices must be in action before attempting to move the patient.
2 If a stretcher is used it must be seen that the head is wholly on it.
3 Bed clothing which has covered the patient in the ward must not be allowed into the operating area. Freshly laundered warmed blankets replace this clothing. In some modern suites even the patient's gown is changed at the transfer area.
4 Lifting and transferring of patients should only be carried out if there are sufficient staff present to do this.

The Patient in the Anaesthetic Room

Note the following points while the patient is in the anaesthetic room.

1 The light must not shine directly into his eyes.
2 Take care of the surroundings when the patient is brought into the operating theatre area. Although all apparatus and requirements should be ready beforehand in the anaesthetic room, the patient should not be able to see any of these preparations.
3 The anaesthetic room should be warm.
4 Noise should be kept to an absolute minimum.
5 Care is taken that a conscious patient cannot view another patient who is perhaps returning from surgery. This of course can be eliminated in theatre suites where there are recovery rooms.
6 Staff must avoid chattering to each other in front of any patient.
7 The patient should be comfortable and warm when waiting in the anaesthetic room. Extra blankets should be available and if his condition permits it extra pillows may make him more comfortable.
8 Limbs should be protected during any movement of the patient.
9 The nurse should assume the responsibility for protecting the patient from unnecessary immodesty or exposure.

It is a very valuable exercise for every Theatre Nurse to lie herself on an Operating Table and on a Patient's Trolley. It is quite amazing to find how narrow these are and how insecure one can feel!

Identification of the Patient

'It is important that the patient is correctly identified.

A correct and accurate operating list is a necessity. It should not be constantly altered. This will avoid bringing the patient to the operating theatre too soon or in the wrong order. It is important that the patient is expected and that there is absolutely no confusion about his presence in the theatre or about his operation.

Children

If a child is being operated on he requires special care in the anaesthetic room. They normally fear strangers and so it is particularly advantageous that the theatre nurse makes friends as soon as possible and preferably has done this, visiting the child in the ward the evening before surgery.

The Patient must never be left unattended at any time in the Theatre for any reason whatsoever.

The Golden Rule in Theatre is always to consider the Patient as one would like oneself or a member of one's family to be considered.

12

What Happens in the Anaesthetic Room?

Preparation of the Anaesthetic Machine

The machine is assembled for use by the anaesthetic room attendant or nurse. The correct circuit is fitted up and the gas supply of nitrous oxide and oxygen is checked.

These gases can be lead from a cylinder supply in which case two cylinders of each must be available on the machine—one in use and one full.

If there is a piped supply of gases from a central store in the hospital it is also important that one cylinder of gas is also available on the machine.

All cylinders must always be checked before the machine is used.

Other equipment necessary is available on the top of the anaesthetic machine. This will include a tested laryngoscope, appropriate sizes of endotracheal tubes, selection of syringes, needles, drugs, skin cleaning material, artery forceps, suction catheter, face mask, and airway.

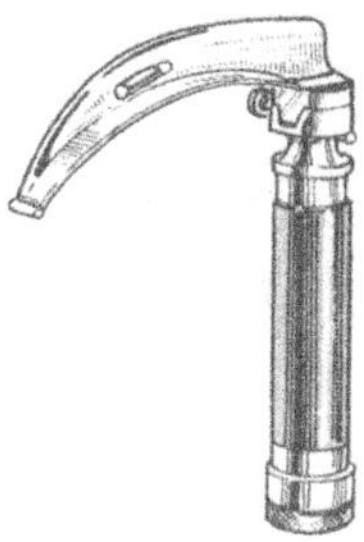

Fig. 5 Laryngoscope

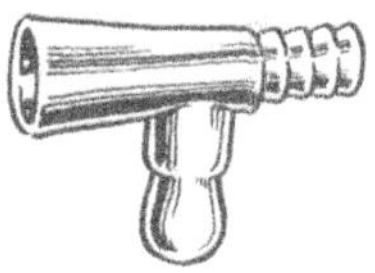

Fig. 6(b) Endotracheal Tube Connection

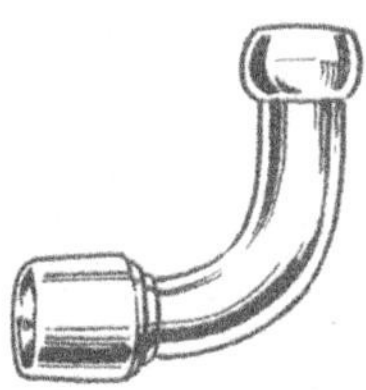

Fig. 6(a) Endotracheal Tube Connection

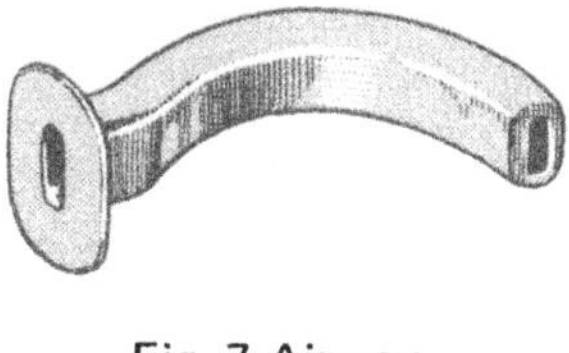

Fig. 7 Airway

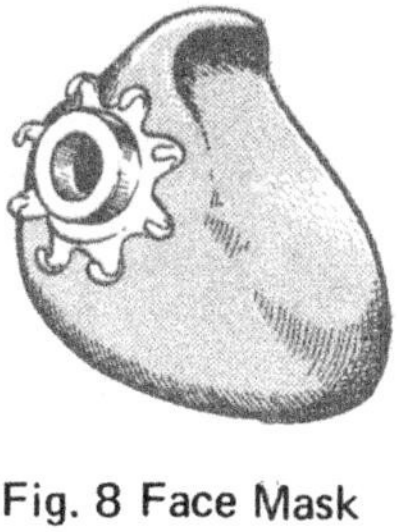

Fig. 8 Face Mask

T

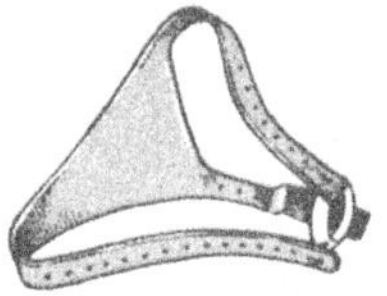

Fig. 9 Anaesthetic Head Harness

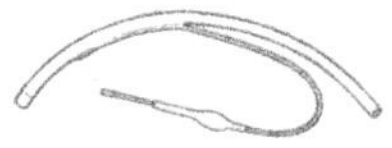

Fig. 10 Endotracheal Tube

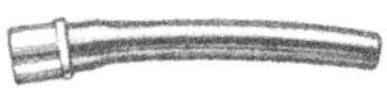

Fig. 11 Anaesthetic Connection

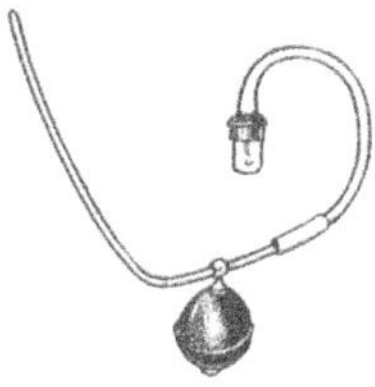

Fig. 12(a) Local Anaesthetic Spray

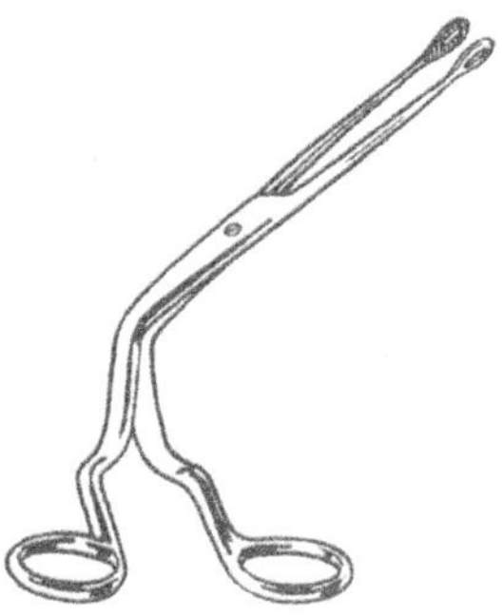

Fig. 13 Laryngeal Forceps

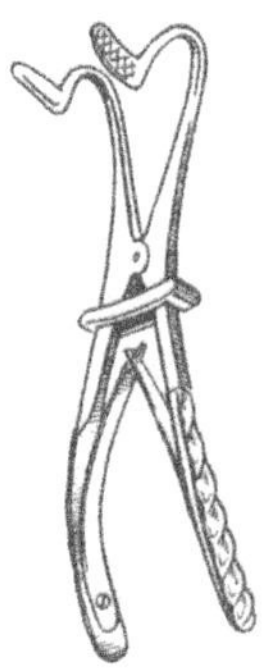

Fig. 14 Mouth Gag

Suction Apparatus

A separate apparatus must be available for anaesthetic use. This must be checked and be in perfect working order before operation. It is important that the tubing and connections are always replaced and ready to connect to the sterile catheter.

It is too late when it is found that a piece is missing.

Induction of the Patient

As stated before the nurse remains with the patient and reassures him or her.

The anaesthetist will arrive and greet the patient by name and also give a few words of reassurance. He will probably have seen the patient in the ward either the evening before or just prior to the pre-medication of the patient.

After the anesthetist has checked the apparatus and machine prepared for him he will draw up the drugs that he will adminster to the patient.

He will ask the nurse to expose a suitable vein by compressing either the forearm or upper arm.

The induction anaesthesia is then given by intravenous injection. The presence of the nurse at this stage beside the patient is of great comfort to him. After the vein has been punctured the anaesthetist will indicate to the nurse that she can release the pressure. This should be done carefully avoiding any movement of the arm or hand. The arm should still be supported.

The anaesthetic agent will rapidly induce the patient. It is important for the nurse to note at this stage that the patient cannot in any way control the action of his limbs and that she is now responsible for protecting the patient from injury.

When the injection is completed the arms must be secured at the patient's sides by using arm rests or alternative means of support.

Never place the patient's hands under the buttocks as severe damage can result from pressure.

Oxygen may be administered by means of a face mask connected to the anaesthetic circuit.

The anaesthetist will then require the laryngoscope and he inserts the endotracheal tube into the trachea. The tube is then inflated and connected to the anaesthetic machine. The tube is then secured.

Other Procedures

Sometimes the procedures that follow may be carried out in other rooms of the theatre suite or actually in the theatre itself. This will vary in each theatre. Individual patients may require specific pre-operative care or investigation. Equipment required for this should be in readiness before the arrival of the patient.

Blood or Fluid Infusion

A drip stand and tray for the procedure is prepared beforehand. Knowledge of the availability of the patient's blood is essential. Care in the identification of the blood is necessary.

Equipment for the transfusion of blood under pressure should be at hand e.g. a Martin pump.

Dressing

All that is necessary is prepared. Wounds of patients returning to theatre or a colostomy stoma may require attention.

Catheterisation

Pre-operatively catheterisation is performed frequently on patients who are about to undergo gynaecological or urological operations.

Oesophagoscopy and Bronchoscopy

Again this can be performed before operation. The suction apparatus and endoscopes must be tested prior to use.

Positioning of the Patients

This is being described later in Chapter 20 pages 56-62.

The Diathermy Pad

This is usually applied before the positioning but never during the anaesthetic induction period.

Aspiration of the Stomach

In emergency surgery a patient may arrive in the anaesthetic room with gastric tube in situ. This will require aspiration. Suction must be available and the attendant ready to lower the patient's head or turn it to one side if required.

Transfer of Patient to the Operating Theatre

The patient is now ready to be transferred to the operating theatre. Staff should know their positions so that the journey is smooth and uneventful. The infusion bottle, the anaesthetic machine, extension of table etc. must be carefully looked after.

13

What are the Most Common Drugs Used in the Anaesthetic Room?

Inhalation Anaesthesia

1 Halothane (Fluothane) — This is non-explosive and quick acting.

2 Ether	This is explosive. It is occasionally used.
3 Cyclopropane	This is explosive. It is well tolerated by the patient and gives rapid induction.
4 Nitrous Oxide	This gas is commonly used combined with oxygen.

Intravenous Anaesthesia

1 Thiopentone Sodium (Pentothal)	This is pleasant and rapid.

Rectal Anaesthesia

1 Bromethol (Avertin) 2 Thiopentone	Both of these drugs can be used in paediatric surgery. It may be given in the ward but always in the presence of an anaesthetist.

Local and Spinal Anaesthesia

1 Lignocaine
2 Procaine

Adrenalin can be added to some local anaesthetic agents. This causes the blood vessels to contract.

Muscle Relaxants, Anti-Relaxants and Secretion Drying Drugs

1 Flaxedil	This is a rapid acting relaxant of shorter duration.

2 Scoline	This is commonly used as a muscle relaxant but must be stored in a refrigerator.
3 Tubarine	The action of this relaxant is of longer duration.
4 Prostigmine	This is an antidote to some muscle relaxants.
5 Atropine	This is used to dry up secretions in the mouth and respiratory tract.

14

What is the Nursing Care of the Patient Having a Local Anaesthetic?

A nurse is always allocated to stay with the patient throughout the administration of a local anaesthetic. The procedure of the injection is explained to the patient. Nurse will also see that the patient is lying as comfortably as possible, is warm enough, and is covered as much as possible.

If the patient is on the operating table the nurse must warn the patient not to move unduly or attempt to turn over as the table is quite narrow.

Quietness must exist. All preparation of the trolley for the operation should have been completed and the trolley covered before the patient is wheeled into theatre. Kidney dishes or trays should be lined with linen to prevent noise when instruments are placed into them.

The nurse who is to be with the patient will sit on a stool beside him, explaining all that is happening and what is required of the patient.

If desired a light cover e.g. swab or towel, may be put over the patient's eyes or his head may be turned to one side.

If any particular position is required care must be taken that the limbs and body are lying comfortably and supported as the operation may take some time. Sometimes the patient will even fall asleep.

The Local Anaesthetic

It must be ascertained from the surgeon the correct strength of local anaesthetic that he would like to use. Great care must be taken that it is known whether adrenalin is added or not. The drug itself must be checked both by the scrub nurse and by the surgeon.

Local anaesthetic must be prepared and checked by the same scrub nurse. It should be discarded if there happens to be a change over of staff.

There are two methods of preparing this anaesthetic with points of safety and asepsis in both methods.

1 The drug is poured into a glass measure on the trolley. (Never a gallipot).
2 The drug is aspirated straight from the bottle by the scrub nurse. The circulation nurse will have first swabbed the top with antiseptic.

Each additional supply of anaesthetic must be checked by the surgeon also. The scrub nurse should always have two syringes in use and always have the other filled even after the initial infiltration has been completed. More may be required.

All sizes of needles should be duplicated and tested immediately before use. The surgeon will use a very fine needle for the first penetration and then progress to both wider and longer needles as he infiltrates the area.

It is most important for all personnel to remember that the patient is awake and can hear all that is being said. This is quite

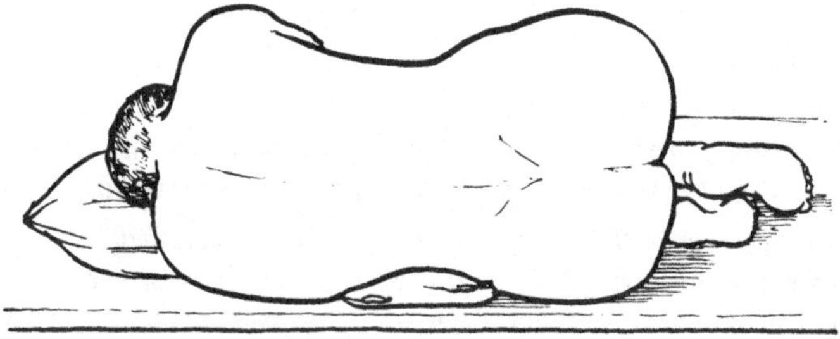

Fig. 15 Left Lateral with Flexed Spine

difficult for staff who are used to having their patients 'asleep'.

Each step is usually described by the surgeon himself or the nurse beside the patient.

The scrub nurse must remember also not to lean on the patient or lay any heavy instrument on the sterile field.

Observation of the patient for any reaction to the anaesthetic agent is most essential.

Assisting at an operation under local anaesthetic is a test of quiet efficiency and the patient will always remember this occasion either as a frightening or a fairly comfortable experience.

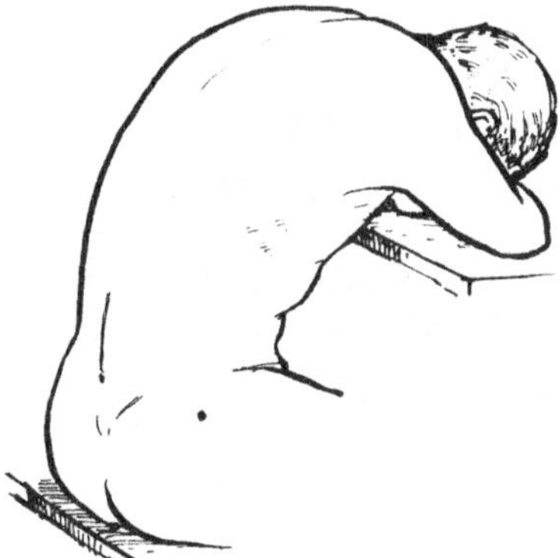

Fig. 16 Sitting on the side of the table with the spine flexed

Spinal Anaesthesia and Epidural Anaesthesia

The same nursing

procedure is carried out. The patient may be in one of two positions.

1 Left lateral with flexed spine.
2 Sitting on the side of the table with the spine flexed.
Support is required from the nurse in this position.

The anaesthetist will carry out this procedure following the same precautions as for local anaesthesia. He will use an aseptic technique wearing sterile gown and gloves. All equipment must be autoclaved in a pack. Care must be taken that drugs are not re-autoclaved.

The patient will require support in assuming a normal position after the procedure. Care is taken that there is no unexpected movement and note that movement is slow at this stage.

15

How Does an Operating List Help the Theatre Nurse in her Work?

A great deal of help and guidance can be gained from a well compiled operating list produced in the theatre the day before.

The Order of the Operating List

This is of prime importance. Change of this order at a later date is both dangerous to the patient and inconvenient to all the staff concerned. There is a great risk of confusion for both the ward and the theatre staff. Of course the theatre staff must be able to adapt adequately and efficiently if the operating list is changed for an emergency situation. This could occur if a patient's condition changed so that surgery was indicated at an earlier stage than was anticipated.

The Content of the List

Patients who have a source of infection are placed at the end of the list. They are never placed first. Certain operations involving areas liable to infection are deferred also e.g. haemorroidectomy.

The Patient's Name

This can sometimes help the nurse to prepare. She may remember this patient as having surgery before and remember useful points about the operation. She can perhaps predict further requirements.

The patient's name could also tell the nurse that he may be from abroad and therefore need especial understanding and assurance if there was a language problem to overcome.

Age of Patient

This is a most important piece of information. The nurse assisting the anaesthetist will want to know this to provide suitable endotracheal tubes, airways, masks etc.

If the patient is a child then again special understanding and help will be required to amuse or placate the child.

The theatre nurse can anticipate special needs or requirements involving instruments because of the age of the patient.

The Condition of the Patient

The patient's medical condition may explain to the theatre

nurse whether the operation is likely to be straightforward or not.

The Operation

This does not always appear on the list as well as the patient's condition. Abbreviations are most confusing to the uninitiated, some are only applicable locally and may be misinterpreted by new or strange staff. Sometimes an operation is referred to as a particular surgeon's operation e.g. Fowler's operation, Cockett's operation.

It is not possible for the theatre nurse to be familar with all these operations but she should know the operations common to her particular theatre or surgeons.

Other indications such as the nature of the operation, the side and site of the operation may be given. In this case special positions may be predicted and the table accessories and fitments checked.

On occasions two teams may operate simultaneously e.g. Synchronous combined abdominal perineal excision of the rectum. The theatre sister would be able to plan the duties of her staff and arrange for extra staff so that the operation will run smoothly. The approach may be shown e.g. vaginal or abdominal.

The Weight of the Patient

This is sometimes given. It may determine the need for longer instruments if the patient is very heavy. If rectal anaesthesia is to be administered the knowledge of the weight is essential to calculate the dosage.

The Ward Number

This is important to the theatre attendant or porter who is going to collect the patient.

The Date and Time of the List

This information should always be clearly and accurately indicated.

The Surgeon's Name and that of his Assistants

These are useful to the theatre staff as specific requirements for the individual surgeon can then be prepared in readiness. Otherwise there may be wastage of material e.g. wrong size of gloves opened, wrong sterile packs etc.

The Anaesthetist's Name

If this is known then the theatre staff will supply his special personal requirements in the way of equipment.

Frozen Section

As far as is predictable when this is required it should be mentioned in the Operation List thus enabling the staff to organise that the specimen will reach the Pathology department with the minimum of delay.

Briefing Staff

If a clear, helpful, and full operation list is provided then the theatre sister can prepare all equipment. She can brief the staff if an intricate operation is scheduled. Duties can be planned in advance. Teaching of staff can be undertaken which gives the nurse an added interest in the following day's list.

All this prior knowledge makes for a smooth-running list.

The Theatre Sister can use the List either as the fortune-teller uses her crystal ball or the detective applies his clues. It depends on the List.

16

What are the Operations to be Performed?

Terminology

It is wise for the theatre nurse to learn the meanings of the commoner terminology used in surgery. They are listed below to help:-

Word Endings

otomy	simple cutting or cutting into e.g. lapar*otomy*—cutting into the abdomen
ostomy	making a hole or opening into e.g. gastr*ostomy*—making an opening into the stomach
ectomy	the removal of e.g. mast*ectomy*—removal of breast
rrhaphy	a suturing or repair e.g. herniorrhaphy—a repair of hernia
desis	a binding or fusion e.g. arthrodesis—a fusion of hip joint
plasty	moulding e.g. tympanoplasty—a plastic operation to the tympanic membrane of the ear
pexy	fastening e.g. nephropexy—fixing of a kidney
oscopy	examination with a lighted instrument e.g. oesophagoscopy—examination of the oesophagus

Procedures

biopsy	removal of tissue for microscopic examination e.g. biopsy of liver
ligation	the tying off of a structure e.g. ligation of varicose veins
dissection	the separation and removal of tissues e.g. dissection of glands of neck
excision	the removal of tissues or a structure e.g. excision of a cyst
anastomosis	the joining up of two structures e.g. anastomosis of bowel

17

What are Some of the Common Operations?

General Surgery

appendicectomy	removal of appendix
cholycystectomy	removal of the gall-bladder
choledochotomy	opening into the common bile duct
partial gastrectomy	removal of part of the stomach
gastro-enterostomy	anastomosis between stomach and jejunum
vagotomy and pyloroplasty	cutting of vagus nerve and refashioning of pylorus
repair of perforation of gastric or duodenal ulcer–self explanatory	
haemorrhoidectomy	removal of haemorrhoids

ligation of varicose veins	tying off of varicose veins
partial thyroidectomy	partial removal of the thyroid gland
resection of small bowel	removal of part of bowel and anastomosis of the two ends
abdominal perineal excision of rectum	this is carried out by two surgeons operating simultaneously in the abdomen and perineum
sympathectomy	excision of a portion of the sympathetic chain
adrenalectomy	removal of one or both adrenal glands

Types of Hernia Repaired at Operation

inguinal
femoral
strangulated
ventral
umbilical

Orthopaedic Surgery

meniscectomy	removal of cartilage from knee
repair of tendon	suturing of tendon
excision of Palmar Fascia	for Dupuytren's disease
osteotomy	cutting into and removing bone
laminectomy	removal of spinal lamina
open reduction and plating of fractures	the bone is exposed and the fracture fixed
synovectomy	removal of diseased capsule of joint

Urological Surgery

cystoscopy	examination of the bladder by cystoscope
cystectomy	removal of bladder and transplant of ureters into colon
uretero-lithotomy	removal of a stone from the ureter
prostatectomy	removal of the prostate gland
nephrectomy	removal of a kidney
cystostomy	opening of the bladder

Ear, Nose and Throat Surgery

tonsillectomy	removal of tonsils
adenoidectomy	curetting and removal of adenoids
trachectomy	opening into trachea in inserting tube
nasal polypectomy	removal of nasal polyps
laryngoscopy	examination of larynx with a laryngoscope
myringotomy	incision of tympanic membrane for the release of pus or fluid
antrostomy	opening into antrum through nose or mouth
simple mastoidectomy	removal of mastoid air cells
stapedectomy	removal of stapes and insertion of prothesis
submucous resection	removal of deflected nasal septum
laryngectomy	removal of larynx

Gynaecological Surgery

hysterectomy	removal of uterus per vagina or abdomen

dilatation and curettage	dilatation of cervical canal and curetting of endometrium
salpinectomy	removal of fallopian tube
colporrhaphy	reconstructive operation of the vagina

Thoracic Surgery

lobectomy	removal of a lobe of the lung
pneumonectomy	removal of the lung
thoracotomy	opening into the chest
valvotomy	opening a valve such as the mitral valve

Vascular Surgery

embolectomy	removal of an embolus
resection of aortic aneurism	excision of aneurysm and inserting a graft

Plastic Surgery

skin grafts	split skin whole skin pedicle
cleft lip and palate	closure of the cleft
rhinoplasty	refashioning of nasal septum

Eye Surgery

iridectomy	removal of iris tissue
corneal graft	removal of part of cornea and insertion of cornea from donor
enucleation	removal of eyeball
cataract operation	extraction of opaque lens of eye

18

How does the Operating Table Function?

Modern operating tables are specifically designed to meet the highly specialised requirements of modern surgery. Modern design has done much to facilitate safe and effective positioning of the patient and to meet the surgeon's needs for accessibility to the part of the body to be operated on.

Familiarity with the movements of the operating table are an essential part of the training of the theatre nurse. It may not always be her duty to position the patient but she may be called upon at any time to alter that position. In addition she will be required to teach other members of staff.

There are many varieties of tables so it is always wise to find out the movements of the particular table in the theatre where you work as soon as possible.

Listed below are the features of a modern theatre table. (See Page 11).

1 It has a locking device to stabilise the table.
2 The length may be adjustable. This is a tremendous advantage if a tall patient requires surgery.
3 The table can be tilted to either side.
4 The top section and the bottom section can be dropped. This is usually a winding movement. If the head needs to be lowered quickly in an emergency this function is very important.
5 There are usually three sections to support the body. This permits flexion or extension of the body parts.
6 There are head extensions e.g. for neurosurgery or endoscopic examination.
7 The foot section may be in two parts. This is

advantageous for some orthopaedic or amputation surgery.

8 X-ray tunnel tops are available which permit the insertion of cassette holders at any position along the table.

In addition there are many accessories and fitments such as chest supports, lithotomy poles, and anaesthetic screen. Those pieces fit into movable clamps on a rail so that they can be in any position, which may be required on the table.

Practically the only specialist table now is the orthopaedic table which is quite different from the table used for all other types of surgery.

Because of this the nurse should familiarise herself with all its intricasies.

Know all the Operating Table movements. Practise when there is no patient on the table till you are familiar with the movements.

19

What are the Protective Measures Taken when Positioning the Patient?

There is no particular way of positioning the patient for a particular operation. The position can vary from patient to patient, surgeon to surgeon, and hospital to hospital.

Positioning however is a most important duty and the nurse can apply her knowledge of the principles of anatomy and physiology.

The aim is to provide the patient with good body alignment. The position is determined by certain points:-

1 the type of operation to be performed

2 the type of anaesthesia to be administered
3 the age, height, weight, and general condition of the patient
4 the location of the lesion or injury
5 the surgical approach

There are certain precautions to observe while positioning the patient. It is important to remember that the patient who has been anaesthetised does not feel any pain and that his limbs must not be forced into any position that would be uncomfortable for him if he were awake.

The Patient's Safety

Constantly this must be the main consideration.

When turning a patient on the operating table always make sure that someone is standing on the opposite side to prevent falling occurring.

The patient should be firmly held after positioning by a strap or straps suitably padded and placed.

Pressure on Nerves

This pressure can result in permanent or temporary paralysis. Always check that there is no pressure.

Pressure on Blood Vessels

Pressure on the blood vessels of limbs can result in thrombosis e.g. no support under the patient's heels to raise the calf of the leg from pressing on the operating table.

Lack of Support of Limbs or Body

No support in the space under the upper arm extended on the arm rest, or in the space in the small of the back is to be avoided. This is particularly important if you are positioning a patient suffering from arthritis or other disability.

Contact of the Patient's Skin

Burns can result when the patient's skin is in contact with metal when the diathermy pad is in place. The skin should always be protected by a covering. A special inspection after positioning is necessary to note that no table fitment or other metal is touching the patient's body.

The Position of the Patient

This must at all stages be fixed and secure. There should be no possibility of any alteration of that state during the operation.

The Proposed Incision Area

This area must be completely accessible to the surgeon with no fitment obstructing his approach.

Transferring of the Patient

It is often possible to save some lifting by seeing that the patient is placed on the operating table mattress in the correct position initially e.g., if the bridge of the table is to be raised then the patient's body should be suitably placed over the bridge.

The Patient's Position during Operation

This position should never be changed without the consent of the anaesthetist. Any sudden movement may cause a sudden drop in blood pressure.

The Patient's Breathing

Care must always be taken to ensure that the patient's breathing is not obstructed by faulty positioning e.g. a pillow obstructing adequate movement of the diaphragm when the patient is lying in the prone position.

Apparatus

Everything likely to be needed should be in readiness and should have been checked for efficiency and completeness before the patient is anaesthetised. Skill is required in the use of equipment. Preparation saves time and temper.

The Patient must look as if he is lying in a comfortable position.

20

What are the More Frequent Positions adopted in the Theatre?

Supine Position

The patient is lying on his back. His arms are secured by his sides with padded arm rests or using a folded towel.

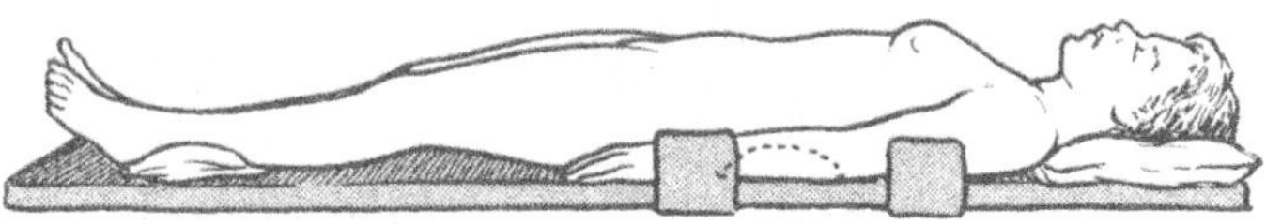

Fig. 17 Supine Position

Alternatively the arms can be placed over the chest and secured by the patient's gown. One arm may be on an arm rest for the easy access of the anaesthetist for infusions. The arm must not be abducted beyond 90° and it must be fixed securely without any pressure.

A support should be in the small of the back and under the ankles.

The patient's legs are uncrossed.

This supine position is used for most abdominal incisions.

Supine Position with Abducted Legs (Fig. 18)

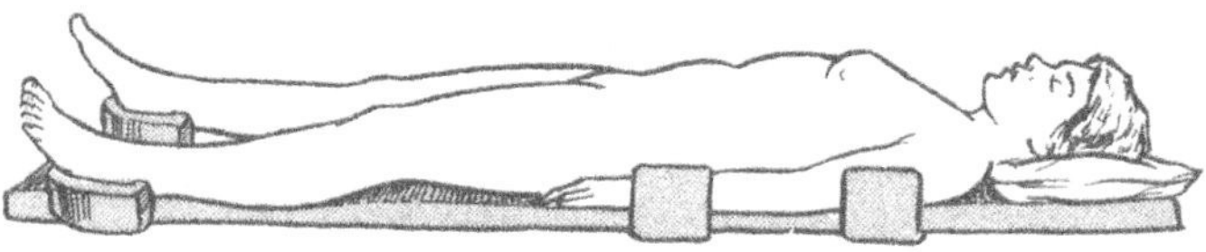

Fig. 18

This position is similar to the supine position described above except that the legs are astride with the heels placed in horse-shoe fitments attached to the foot of the table or placed on a padded board.

This position is used mainly for operations on varicose veins.

Supine Position with Neck Extended (Fig. 19)

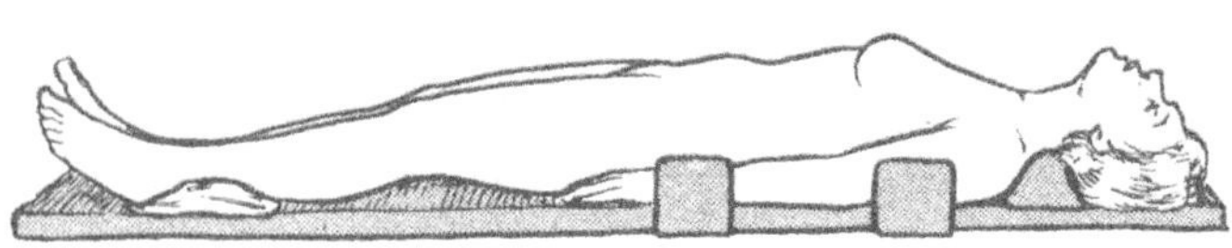

Fig. 19

Again the basic supine position is adopted. The head is

extended by placing it on a padded rest at the head of the table. This may sometimes be lowered.

Sometimes a pad is placed under the shoulders and the head is resting on a small pillow. The head may also be turned to one side.

This position is adopted for operations on the trachea and the thyroid gland.

Gall-Bladder Operation Position (Fig. 20)

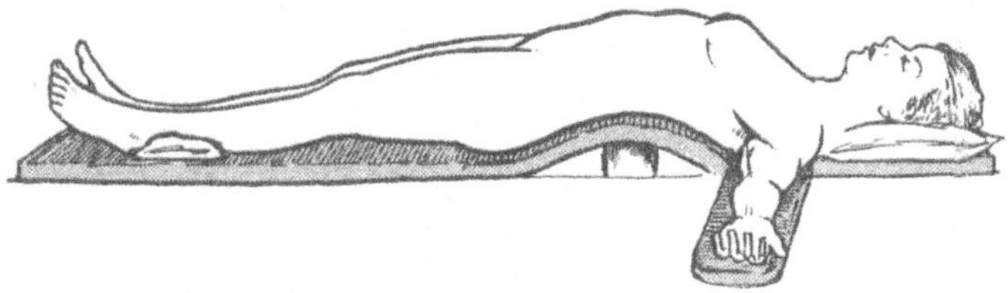

Fig. 20

The patient is positioned over the bridge with the costal margin at the level of the elevator.

Prone Position (Fig. 21)

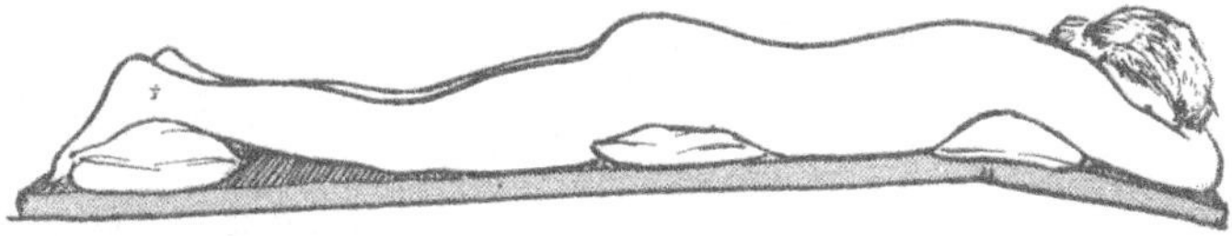

Fig. 21

This requires efficient teamwork. First the patient is turned into the lateral position and then on to his face. Pillows are placed before turning–positioned under the shoulders, pelvis, and ankles. The anaesthetist will usually care for the patient's head. Toes must be free from pressure and adequate free movement must be allowed for lower ribs and diaphragm. The head of the table is dropped slightly to secure a more comfortable position. Great care must be taken of the arms in this positioning. They are secured in front of the face. Operations on the back require this position.

Lithotomy Position

The buttocks are placed at the break of the lower section of the table when the patient is being transferred. Both legs are supported at this stage. The padded stirrup poles are both in position at the same level. Simultaneously each leg is flexed and the feet are put into the slings—one loop around the sole and the other around the ankle. It is important that the legs are raised and lowered at the same time. This procedure must be carried out with slow and deliberate movements by two people. Care is taken that there is no popliteal pressure. The bottom of the table is lowered. The buttocks will extend beyond the table slightly. (Sometimes a sandbag will be placed under the buttocks). This position is used for operations with a rectal, perineal, and vaginal approach.

Trendelenberg Position

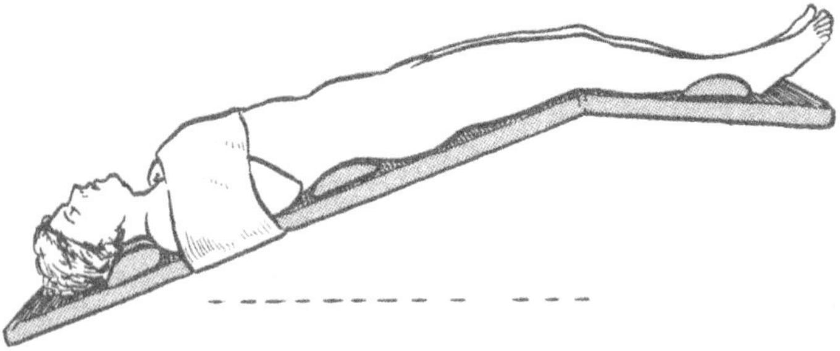

Fig. 22 Trendelenberg Position

The patient should be lying on the corrugated mattress. The table is altered to lower the head and body, and to flex the knees a little.

If shoulder rests are used care must be taken that they are well placed and padded and fitted securely on the outer parts of the shoulders thus avoiding the nerves of the brachial plexus.

When restoring the position the legs are straightened first.

This position is used on operations in the pelvic cavity to allow better exposure by allowing the intestines to fall away from the operation site.

Combined Trendelenberg and Lithotomy Position

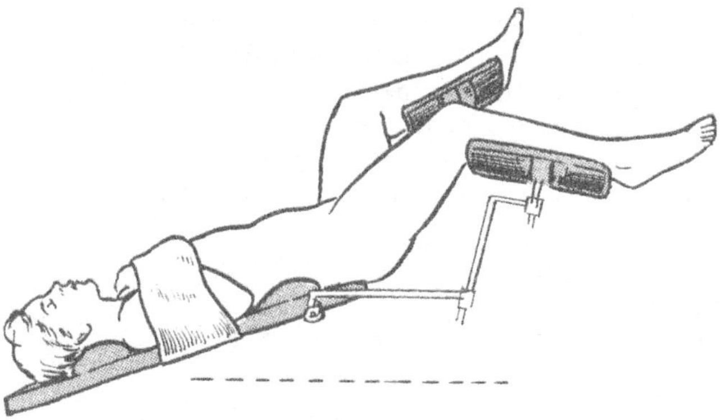

Fig. 23 Combined Trendelenberg and Lithotomy Position

The legs are placed and fixed in the Lloyd Davis Stirrups. The table is altered to the Trendelberg position. The bottom of the table is dropped. The buttocks are slightly projecting beyond the table.

This position is used for synchronous combined excision of the rectum.

Lateral Position (Fig. 24)

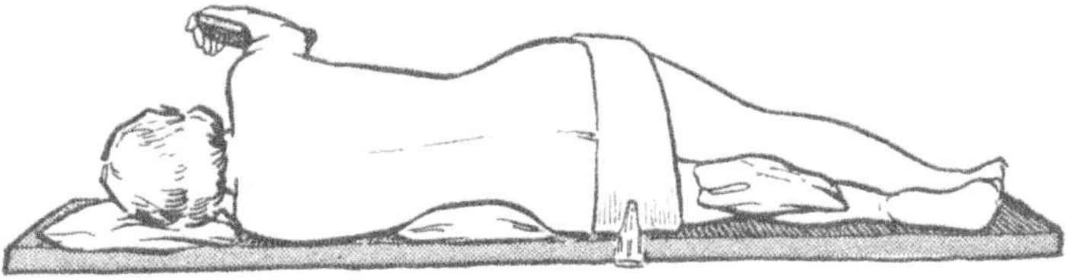

Fig. 24

This position requires teamwork. The affected side is uppermost. The patient is on his side and his hips are brought back to the edge of the table.

A pillow is placed between his legs with the lower leg flexed and the upper leg straight. Another small cushion is sometimes placed under his ankles.

A chest and pelvic support may be used to keep the patient over with the shoulders level with the hips.

The upper arm is supported and secured on a padded arm rest.

A padded strap is placed round the hips and under the table.

The table may be flexed slightly or tilted.

This position is used for most chest operations.

Flexed Lateral Position

This is similar to the lateral position which has been described but the table is broken to spread apart the space between the lower ribs and pelvis.

The table will be straightened before closure.

This gives the surgeon good access and is usually used in kidney operations.

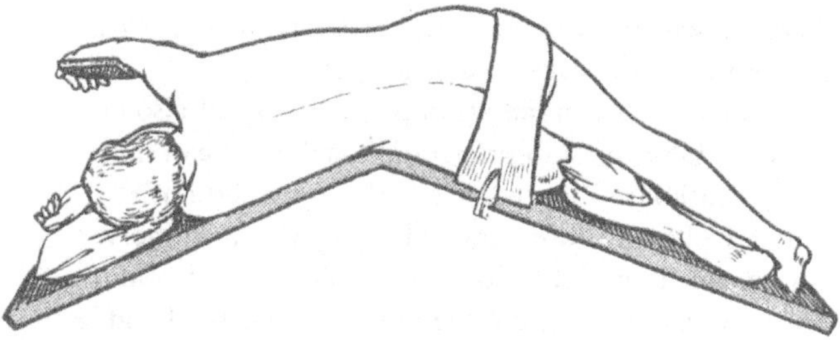

Fig. 25 Flexed Lateral Position

Neurosurgical Positions

The head of the table is removed and the patient's head is placed in a padded head rest.

There is also sitting position for neurosurgery with a special fitment to support the patient.

The arms are flexed across the abdomen and allowed to rest on a pillow in the patient's lap.

21

How is the Patient's Skin Prepared Before Operation?

The patient's skin may be prepared either in the ward or in the operating theatre. There are advantages in carrying out this preparation in both situations.

Time of Preparation

The procedure may be embarrassing or uncomfortable to

the patient. In the case of an emergency where the patient may be in great pain then it would be advisable that this is carried out after the patient is anaesthetised.

The timing of the preparation procedure must also be noted. Generally the skin preparation is done the evening before operation in the ward area. There are certain advantages when it is done immediately prior to surgery. Better lighting is available, and bacteriologically it is more satisfactory in the operating theatre. On the other hand the operation time and the anaesthetic time are being prolonged. There is also the presence of loose hairs to be taken into consideration.

The Purpose of Skin Preparation

Before surgery this makes the skin clean and as free from bacteria as possible. This should be achieved without causing irritation or damage to the skin surface. It is impossible of course to render the skin sterile but by the removal of hair and the use of antiseptic lotions or soap the skin is made as clean as possible.

The Areas to be Prepared

The areas to be prepared must be examined and a note made of any abnormal lesion or reaction. If any is noted it should be reported to the surgeon immediately for his further instructions.

The extent of the area to be shaved is determined by the site of the incision. A generous area must be shaved and prepared thus reducing the danger of contamination to the skin around the wound area. Skin folds must be stretched so that the complete area is cleaned.

The umbilica must have careful attention by using a

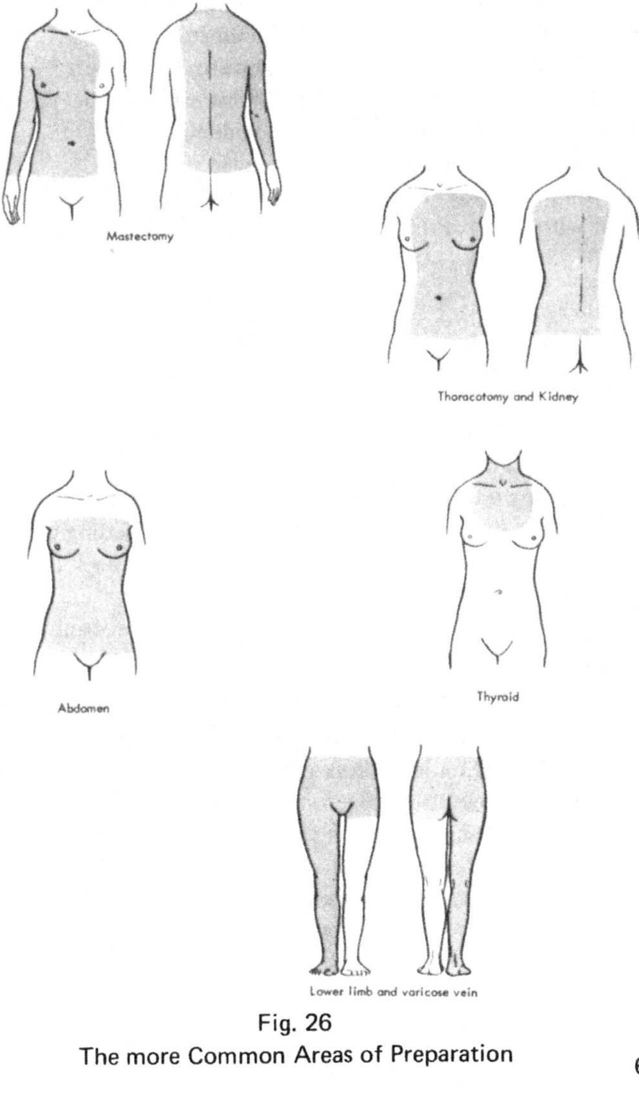

Fig. 26
The more Common Areas of Preparation

cotton tipped applicator if necessary. A mild antiseptic may be applied after the shave and the area blotted dry.

The patient is left comfortable and warm.

This procedure must not be carried out in a great hurry. It can be a distressing experience for the patient if it is not explained to the patient all that is entailed.

It is very important for the theatre nurse to familiarise herself with the areas to be prepared for each operation.

22

How is the Patient's Skin Prepared at Operation?

The skin surface necessary for the operation is exposed by the circulating nurse. She must avoid unnecessary movement or flapping of the sheets covering the patient by folding them down neatly and making sure that no part will fall back over the exposed area.

The actual skin cleaning may be done in two ways and carried out by either the scrub nurse or the surgeon.

1 before scrubbing
2 after donning gloves and gown

The surgeon or nurse will take the tray containing sponge-holding forceps mounted with foam sponges or swabs, and a skin cleaning lotion. The skin is prepared starting at the incision site moving outwards and in a circular motion taking care not to return to the original site. This sponge-holder and sponge are discarded. This procedure is repeated with fresh sponge-holders and sponges until the operator is satisfied that the whole area has been covered adequately

Particular attention must be paid to the umbilicus and any folded area in the skin.

The process will vary depending on the area e.g. preparing a leg or a vaginal area. The unsterile personnel should be ready to assist if lifting of the limb is required.

Particular note must be taken that no fluid is allowed to form a pool under the patient as this may be the cause of a burn if diathermy is used.

The antiseptic may or may not contain a colouring agent.

Usually an area larger than that needed is prepared in case the surgeon has to extend the incision.

If this procedure is carried out when nurse is wearing a sterile gown and gloves great care must be taken that the fluid is not allowed to run up the sponge-holder or that the sponge-holder is held too far down thus contaminating the user's gloves. It is also important that there is no contamination of the operator's gown by touching any unsterile material or equipment.

The sponge-holders are returned to the tray and not handed to the circulating nurse. They are then removed from the area to be cleared away.

Two separate trays should be available if two areas are to be prepared e.g. the donor area for a skin graft procedure and the operation site itself.

Frequently in gynaecological surgery the vaginal and abdominal areas are both prepared.

A very mild antiseptic is used when preparing the skin for areas around the eyes, nose, ears, and face.

Traumatic Injuries

These are treated in a different manner. They commonly involve a hand or a foot. A quantity of solution of Cetavlon 10% or a similar mild lotion is prepared in a basin along with a sterile sponge and sometimes a nail brush.

The injured part—if at all practicable—is placed in this

basin or if not practicable on a waterproof sheet. Any dirt or grit can then be removed and the injured part made ready for operation.

Following adequate preparation of the site the patient is ready for draping

23 How is the Patient Draped at Operation?

This is an important stage of the operation and the draping can vary greatly. Each draping technique must provide an effective barrier so that the area for placing sterile instruments and hands is completely sterile.

The whole patient's body and the operating table should be completely covered by sterile towels.

Draping may be carried out by the scrub nurse or more generally by the surgeon. The scrub nurse and surgeon both wear sterile gowns and sterile gloves.

Folding of the Drapes

Folding of drapes prior to packing can save time and make for ease and safety at the start of the operation. Certain factors must be observed during this procedure.

1 The towels and sheets should be prepared on the trolley by the scrub nurse in the order that they are required.

2 The sterile gloves of the operator should always be protected by holding a towel under a cuff of material.

3 Each article must be handed carefully to the surgeon

by the scrub nurse in such a way that neither she nor the surgeon contaminate their gloves in any way.

4 The towel or sheet should also be handed in such a way that no extra handling is required by the surgeon.

5 No towel or sheet should be handed over an unsterile area or surface.

6 If a drape is incorrectly placed it must be discarded.

7* It is essential that the area below and perhaps above the incision is protected by a waterproof sheet. This sheet is usually of a disposable material these days.

8* If a Mayo table is brought over the operating table this also must be protected by a piece of waterproof sheeting.

*Both these areas are liable to dampness and consquently open to contamination from the patient's unsterile covering underneath.

9 Towel clips can be fixed under the flap of the towel. This keeps them out of the way of the surgeon. Alternatively towels can be sutured on.

10 A towel clip fixed through the drapes has its points contaminated and therefore if it is removed for any reason it must be discarded immediately.

11 Drapes may be coloured. This will reduce the glare and eye strain for the operating team.

Draping of the Operation Area

There are many varieties of sterile plastic film coverings for the actual incision area. This prevents any danger of the surgeon handling the patient's skin with his sterile gloved hands.

This film is either self adherent to the skin or a spray is used first before the film is applied. Designs of this plastic film are available to cover almost all incision sites.

The drapes can be applied before the rest of the towels but it is equally often done after they are in position.

The plastic film coverings also obviate the need for skin towels to be used on the skin edges after the incision is made.

Draping of the Mayo Stand

A folded tray cover—similar to a domestic pillow cover—is slipped over the stand. The hands of the scrub nurse are protected by a cuff. She must stand well back during the procedure. The cover is then allowed to unfold over the support of the stand.

Basic Draping Routines—Abdominal Incision Draping

1 The waterproof sheeting and first towel are usually applied first to the area over the lower abdomen.
2 The opposite towel is applied.
3 The towel for the side facing the surgeon is then handed, and immediately followed up with two towel clips.
4 The fourth is then applied with another two towel clips.
5 The top and bottom of the sterile field is then completely draped with two large sheets. The surgeon will receive the short end of this sheet at the opposite side of the table from the nurse. It is important that the unfolding of this sheet is carefully done and over the already covered area and that no part is allowed to drop.
6 The top sheet is allowed to fall over the anaesthetic screen giving the anaesthetist access to the patient's head.
7 If the whole of the operating table is not covered with a good over flap then additional sheets must be used.

8 If an armboard is in position a towel is used to cover this area.

Basic Draping Routines—Limb Draping

1 The limb is held by a circulating member of staff while the surgeon cleans the skin.
2 A waterproof sheet and a towel or sheet are then placed under the limb.
3 The limb is then laid into a sterile drape wrapped completely and fastened securely by a clip or bandage.
3a Alternatively material such as stockinette is prepared and may be unrolled to cover the limb. The incision area of course determines which of these procedures is adopted.
4 The operating table area is then completely draped.

Basic Draping Routines—Head or Neck Draping

This draping may vary considerably but one common method is as follows:-

1 The scrub nurse to prepare one waterproof sheet and one towel and lay them together.
2 These are placed under the patient's head while it is being held.
3 Immediately a towel folded into a triangle is placed on top.

This procedure can be done in one movement by having the three towels prepared in this fashion.

4 The corners of the triangle are then folded up over the patient's forehead or required site and secured by a towel clip.
5 A waterproof sheet and towel are placed over the patient's chest to meet the other drapes.

6 The operating table area is then completely covered.
7 An additional sheet can be clipped up to the drip stands to allow both the surgeon and the anesthetist freedom of movement.

Basic Draping Routines—Lithotomy Draping

1 A waterproof sheet and towel are laid together and placed under the patient's buttocks.
2 Two leggings are manoeuvred over the legs positioned in the stirrups.
3 A sheet with an opening is then placed over the perineal area.
4 Towel clips are then used to hold the sheet in position around the incision site.

Every effort must be made to isolate the wound from any bacterial contamination. Draping–which should be supervised by the surgeon–well done and in a routine fashion, can save much time and perhaps inconvenience at a later period of the operation.

24
What are the Common Incisions?

1 Iliac Incision

This is used for inguinal hernia operations.

2 Right Grid-Iron Incision

The incision is at McBurney's point and is used for the operation for the removal of the appendix.

3 Right and Left Upper Paramedian Incision and Upper Mid-line Incision

These incisions are used for abdominal operations including stomach, gall-bladder, duodenum, etc.

4 Right and Left Lower Paramedian Incisions and Lower Mid-line Incision

These are used for gynaecological and urological operations.

5 Transverse Elipse Incision

This is used for the repair of umbilical hernia.

6 Kocher's Incision (Sub-costal)

This is used for gall-bladder operations and the incision of sub-phrenic abcess.

7 Sternotomy or Sternal Incision

This is an incision through the sternum for open-heart surgery.

8 Thoraco-Abdominal Incision

This is used for total gastrectomy and chest surgery.

Collar Incision

This is used for sub-total and total removal of the thyroid gland.

Lumbar Incision

This is used for kidney operations.

There are of course many other incisions allied to the particular surgeries. The theatre nurse will become more familar with those as she gains more experience. The common incisions above give a guide to the nurse—especially for the draping technique. Incisions can vary with the surgeon or operation.

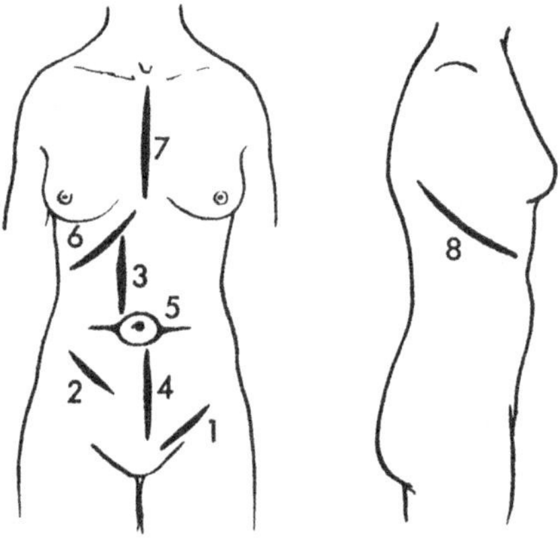

1 Inguinal
2 Appendix
3 Paramedian
4 Mid-line
5 Transverse
6 Costal
7 Sternal
8 Thoraco-abdominal

Fig. 27

25

How does the Theatre Nurse Work the Diathermy Machine?

Application of Diathermy

This is normally considered a nursing duty.

Understanding the machine is essential to the practical nurse working in the operating theatre.

The Diathermy Machine's Purpose

The machine is to provide for the surgeon electro-coagulation to seal off blood vessels and cut or cauterise tissue. Two electrodes are required, an active one for the surgeon's use and an indifferent electrode (the pad) applied to the surface of the patient's body. Both electrodes are connected to the machine.

In up-to-date machines it is impossible to connect these up incorrectly as the two fittings are quite different—but there may still be some older machines around.

Flexes should be long enough to reach the patient and the operating site. Avoid any need for pulling or straining as this could result in the disconnection or the loosening of the wire.

The lead and diathermy point that the surgeon uses are sterilised along with the other instruments and the end of the lead is handed to the circulating nurse by the scrub nurse so that she may connect it before the operation begins. The foot pedal is positioned near the surgeon.

The power is regulated by control knobs either for cutting or coagulating current. Activation only occurs when the foot pedal is pressed.

The Indifferent Electrode

Usually this electrode is a lead pad with the cable attachment. If the cable is not moulded on to the pad care must be taken that the pad and cable are firm and secure. Any wrinkling or ridging must be ironed out.

Recently an electrode intended for use at one operation and then discarded has been introduced.

Methods of Application

1 A pocket of lint made with sixteen thicknesses and with

an area two inches larger than the lead pad all around should be available for each pad. This is saturated with a 20% solution of isotonic saline. This pocket is wrung out before insertion of the pad. It is important that the lead pad is completely covered.

A bandage is required to keep it in place when it is applied.

2 Another method is to apply a saline cream directly to the lead pad. It is essential that the cream covers the pad completely.

The pad is then applied by using a bandage or other means of firm support.

3 A foil disposable pad and cable can be applied without cream to the patient's skin. It can be fixed with adhesive.

Sites of Application

The pad is usually applied to the side opposite to that of the proposed operation.

1 the outer aspect of the thigh
2 placed under the buttock

Application of the Pad

The site is chosen, the apparatus is prepared, and the nurse applies the pad. The pad is never applied to a bony surface or over a previous scar but to a fleshy part of the patient's body.

Firm pressure is essential for good contact.

As a rule the electrode is applied in the anaesthetic room. However, it should never be done before or during the induction of the anaesthetic.

Other Points to Remember

1 Diathermy should never be used if an explosive gas e.g. ether, is being used by the anaesthetist.
2 The scrub nurse must also be careful during the use of diathermy that the point or pencil is kept in a quiver made of insulating material. Accidental operation of the foot pedal could cause burning of the patient if the diathermy point is left on the operation site unguarded.
3 At the end of the operation when the pad is removed the nurse must always examine the skin carefully before the patient returns to the ward.
4 If there is anything abnormal this must be reported immediately.

Only suitably Trained Staff should be involved in the application of Diathermy.

26

How are the Packets Opened by the Circulating Nurse?

There are a variety of opening techniques according to the method of packing or sterilisation of articles used in the theatre.

Before opening any pack the nurse must check certain points:-

1 That the contents of the pack is really what she wants or has been asked for.
2 That the sterilising date has not expired.
3 That the outer wrap is intact.
4 That the sterilising test tape is suitably changed.

There are three main types of packs to be opened.

1 The large pack to be opened on to a trolley.
2 The smaller supplementary pack that the circulating nurse opens for the scrub nurse.
3 The peel pack.

The Large Pack

This can be the basic operation pack with the required drapes and swabs. It has usually a dust cover, such as a paper or polythene bag.

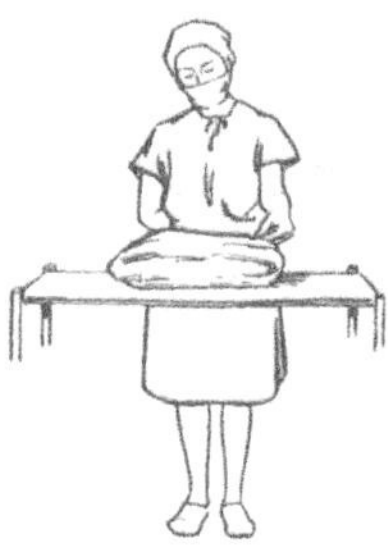

Fig. 28

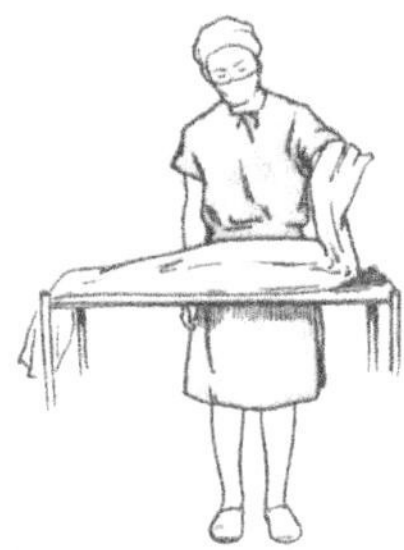

Fig. 29

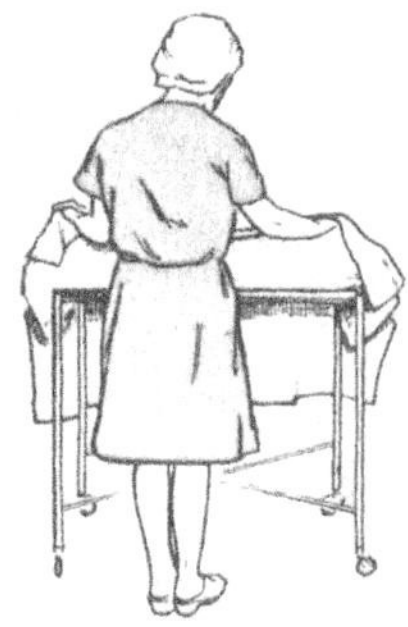

Fig. 30

1 The pack is removed first from the bag and placed on a clean theatre instrument trolley. (Fig. 28).
2 The circulating nurse will remove the autoclave tape discarding it before proceeding any further.
3 Standing in front of the trolley the side pieces of the outer wrapping are folded down over the sides of the trolley. (Fig. 29).
4 Then the hands are placed under the fold of the pack and unfolded back over the edge of the front of the trolley. (Fig. 30).

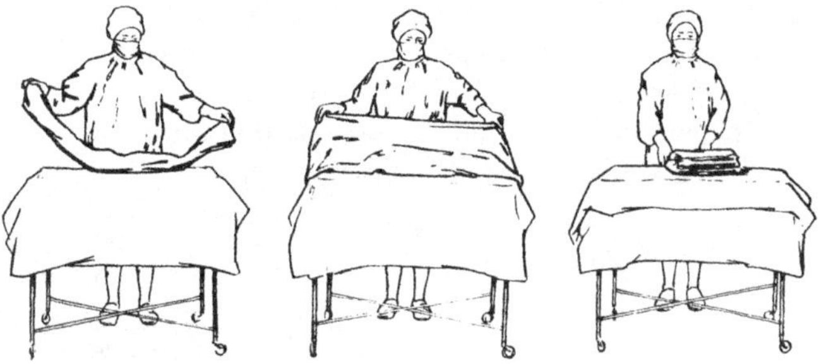

Fig. 31 Fig. 32 Fig. 33

5 The circulating nurse then goes round to the other side of the trolley and repeats these moves. (Figs. 31-33).

It is important that the circulating nurse does not lean over the inner wrap to unfold the other side. She must avoid any extra handling of the pack and allow plenty of room for unfolding.

There may be a colour code on the outer and inner wraps e.g. white for outer and green for inner.

The Supplementary Pack

This is usually handled by the circulating nurse.

1 The outer dust cover is removed.
2 The pack is taken out and the bag discarded.
3 The packet will have been packed in the envelope fashion or the one described above for the large pack.

The Envelope Type Pack

The circulating nurse will state what the article is before opening the pack.

1 The autoclave tape is removed and discarded.
2 Holding the pack in one hand the open end is pulled down and away from the nurse.
3 The packet is unfolded making sure that the open end is always away from the opener.

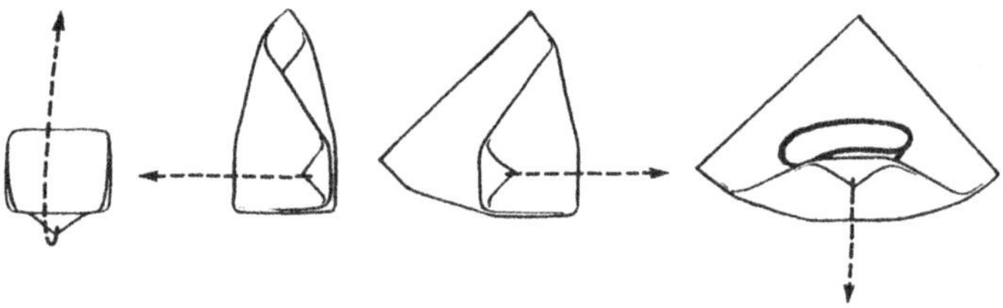

Fig. 34 Envelope Pack Opening

4 The side flaps are then unfolded firmly and with a downward movement leaving the packed article available for the scrub nurse to handle.
5 The circulating nurse should stand well back from the trolley and take care not to touch anything or anyone during this procedure of unfolding.

The Peel Pack

Sometimes there is a very thin line between the sterile and the non-sterile. This is so with the Peel Pack. Great care should be taken to open both sides at the same time so that a smooth movement is achieved. The scrub nurse will pick up the article in between. If there is any doubt that there has been contamination of the contents the packet should be discarded.

Any break in aseptic procedure can result in a longer stay in hospital as a result of sepsis.

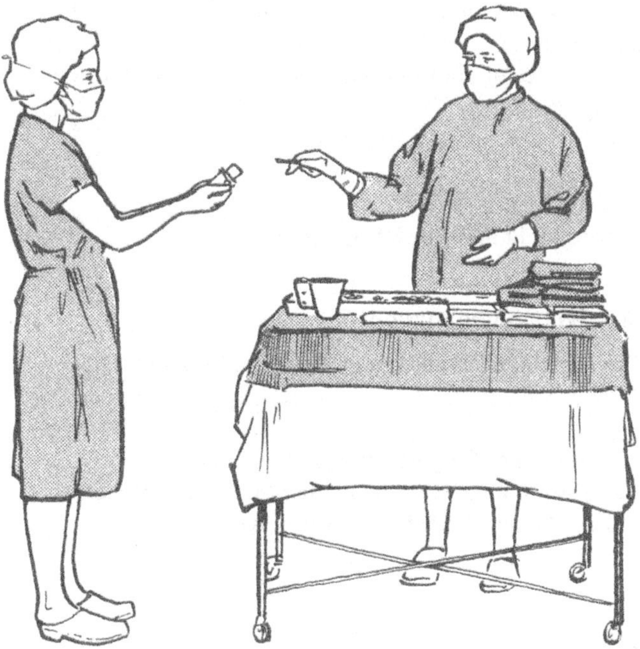

Fig. 35 Peel Pack

Other Wraps

Any other type of wrap or container may need special precautions.

There are too many different versions to go into detail here. The nurse is therefore advised to check with a strange type of packing before proceeding. The same principles will apply of course as above.

The nurse should of course make sure that she knows how to open all packets in the operating theatre to which she is assigned. It is not good practise to leave this to the time of operation when time can be an all important factor for the patient's welfare.

The practice of emptying on to a sterile field is not to be encouraged.

Trolleys

These should never be left unattended.

Sources of Contamination

The nurse must at all times be alert to the sources of contamination.

Practice makes for perfection and quickness. Contamination must stop the moment it occurs. Packets should not be opened before it is necessary.

27

How is the Swab, Instrument, and Needle Count Conducted?

Each operating department should have an agreed policy and a definite written code of practice. All members of the team must co-operate and follow this code of practice with absolutely no deviation.

With the introduction of more and more Central Sterile Supply Departments the variety of swabs is becoming less and consequently there is less confusion. Here are a few general rules adhered to in many operating suites.

Colour Identification

Green swabs for anaesthetic use only.

Blue or other colour swabs are used for skin cleaning purposes or as a dressing after operation.

Raytex swabs should be used for all operations however trivial the operation may be. These swabs have a barium sulphate thread through the swab. This thread is easily detectable on X-ray. All sizes of swabs—from the very tiny pledget to the large abdominal pack—are available with this raytex thread. Raytex swabs are always made up in multiples of five.

Points to Remember during the Swab Count

Some form of chinagraph board or sheet of paper is used in the operating theatre for recording purposes.

The number of the various types of swab in use for the operation is recorded here.

The scrub nurse will check all the swabs to be used separately and audibly in the presence of the circulating nurse.

If there is a discrepancy in a bundle the entire bundle should be removed from the theatre.

A discarded swab from the operation field must be picked up carefully, opened out, and hung on the swab rack immediately so that the scrub nurse can check the swab count at any time during the operation.

Care should be taken by all concerned that no swab is attached to any specimen being removed from the operation site.

At no time must any swab be removed from the theatre during an operation. The scrub nurse must be alert to the number of swabs in use at the wound site at any one time and control this number. She should also note if any swab is tucked inside the wound.

Small swabs should not be used inside a cavity unless they are mounted on a sponge holder.

A complete count is carried out before a cavity is to be closed and the nurse must inform the surgeon accordingly. An additional check is made during insertion of skin sutures.

The circulating nurse must ascertain that all swabs are removed from the theatre after the operation.

Number of Counts of Swabs

1 when the bundle is prepared.
2 when the scrub nurse checks at operation with the circulating nurse.
3 before the cavity is closed.
4 before the skin sutures are completed.

Instruments

The check of instruments used for one operation will vary according to the method of preparing the instruments. The essential point is that the scrub nurse must be aware of all the instruments on her tray or trolley:-

1 before the operation.
2 prior to the closure of the cavity.
3 when the tray or trolley is being cleared away.

If a pre-set tray system is in operation this can make the control of the instrument count easier. These trays are composed of basic sets of instruments.

Instruments with screws should be checked before handing them to and receiving from the operator and of course again after cleaning.

Instruments with teeth and fine hooks should also be examined in the same way.

Needles

By a similar procedure the scrub nurse should make a count of all needles in use. This can be recorded with the swab count.

In the same way as she controlled the swab count at the wound area so should she control the needles.

This will mean parting only with a needle as another one is returned. Examination of the needle should also be made to be sure the needle is intact.

It is essential during this complete count routine that the surgeon co-operates and allows adequate time for the count to be carried out.

Any irregularity however trivial should always be reported to a Senior Nurse in order to safeguard both the Patient and the Nurse.

28

How are Specimens Cared for by the Theatre Nurse?

There is no room for doubt or guesswork in carrying out the procedure for the care of the specimen. No nurse would like to be in the position of a patient being told by the surgeon that the specimen of tissue removed has been lost and that the operation has been in vain.

Carelessness or lack of routine is always to blame when this happens.

Equipment Required

The equipment required will vary from hospital to hospital

and you should therefore familiarise yourself with the routine of the theatre and laboratory staff where you are working.

Routine Specimens

1 For a Culture

A throat swab. This is a test-tube sterilised with a wool-tipped stick. It is used for serum or pus exudate.

2 For a Large Specimen

A clean container which can be a bag, a glass jar (with a lid), or a plastic container (preferably opaque) of a suitable size.

3 For a Small Specimen

A small glass container with a screwtop or lid–usually sterilised.

Labelling System

It is also necessary to have a standard labelling system which will record:-

1 the patient's name
2 the ward number
3 the date of operation
4 the nature of the specimen

Nursing Procedure

The scrub nurse receives the specimen either directly–as in the case of the culture swab or small biopsy–into the sterile bottle or into a sterile dish on her trolley.

A patient may have more than one specimen taken.

Each specimen is taken separately and placed in a separate container and labelled accordingly.

The scrub nurse then hands the specimen to a circulating nurse telling her explicitly the nature of the specimen.

The circulating nurse must deal promptly with the specimen.

The specimen now in its container is prepared for transfer to the pathological department. Formalin 10% must not be added unless the operator requests this. The circulating nurse will then complete the label for the container with the relevant information (see page 86).

She should carry this whole procedure out with as few interruptions as possible and always before that particular patient leaves the operating theatre.

At the end of the operation the pathology form will be completed by one of the medical staff.

The specimen suitably labelled and complete with its form is then placed ready for collection.

Sometimes a record is kept of the specimens sent. This is checked by the messenger and again the pathology department.

Culture Specimens

These specimens must not be allowed to lie for any length of time and should be sent to the appropriate laboratory immediately.

Frozen Sections

The pathology department are informed of the operation involving a frozen section specimen. Immediately the biopsy is removed by the surgeon it is taken to the pathologist. In some modern theatre suites a laboratory for this purpose may be available.

The pathology form will have been completed before the start of the operation. It is very important that the message from the pathology department is taken carefully—and preferably—by a member of the medical staff.

In some suites a direct communication systèm is available between the pathology department and the theatre. The surgeon in this instance can speak to the pathologist himself. This is a very satisfactory arrangement where it exists.

Fluids

Fluids must be measured accurately and the amount recorded. The surgeon will advise on the amount to be kept for examination.

No tissue should be discarded unless after specific instruction.

29
What are Some of the Duties of the Circulating Nurse?

A good circulating nurse anticipates the needs of the scrub nurse. This position is really a most important one in the operating theatre.

The circulating nurse must have her eyes everywhere, her ears wide open, and be able to foresee the needs of the whole operating team.

A good circulating nurse should pride herself on having all materials, sutures, and equipment available before the scrub nurse requires it. Efficiency only comes with experience working with the same team. The circulating nurse is every bit as important as the scrub nurse.

The experienced circulating nurse expects the unexpected! She is also able to produce articles not anticipated very quickly. She herself is familiar with the storage of all items in the operating theatre.

She also knows how and where to summon help if this is required knowing the experience and ability of all staff.

The site of the emergency equipment is also another thing with which she must make herself familiar.

There is usually a definite area in the operating theatre that is restricted to 'scrubbed' personnel. The circulating nurse does not enter this area and also restricts any other staff members from doing so.

The circulating nurse and the scrub nurse work together as a team, in very close co-ordination with each other from the preparations for the operation to its completion.

The theatre nurse should be instructed, guided, and supervised in the circulating duties until she is entirely proficient and confident to carry these duties out.

Her movements must always be quiet and deliberate. She should never turn sharply or turn her back on any sterile field. She must never lean over sterile material or leave the theatre with no nurse present.

Knowledge of the individual preferences of surgeons should be known by her.

Many of the circulating nurse's duties have already been described in detail. However here are some more procedures to help the nurse tackle any difficulty that may arise during her time in theatre.

Preparation of the Instrument Trolley

This is done in complete co-ordination with the scrub nurse. A certain routine will be followed in each theatre.

The circulating nurse should consult the operating card on all the routine instruments required for the particular operation.

The Mayo table and any other furniture necessary is placed in the position suitable for the scrub nurse.

The Preparation of the Patient

The circulating nurse receives the patient and helps to position the table and other apparatus. Finishing touches to the position of the patient may be carried out. The patient is then prepared by turning the coverings down and exposing the incision site.

A final check is made that there is no metal touching the patient's skin or any other fault in the positioning.

The Theatre Equipment

1 The kick-buckets are placed in position usually on the right hand side of each operator. The scrub nurse also has one at her disposal.
2 The diathermy machine and the suction apparatus are placed near the field of operation and the circulating nurse awaits the sterile leads in order to connect them up to both pieces of equipment.
3 The footplate of the diathermy machine should be placed at a spot suitable for the surgeon.
4 Platforms may be required for some members of the operating team.
5 The operating light is also focussed on the incision area. Maybe a mobile light will also be required.

Gowning of the Personnel

The circulating nurse must be in constant attendance at this stage providing gloves for each person and tying gowns. The circulating nurse reaches inside the donned gown and grasps the sleeve seam pulling the gown on gently. It is then fastened by the method employed—the technique will vary according to the style of the gown.

Moving Sterile Equipment

The circulating nurse will be asked to move trolleys, basin stands, and the Mayo table. She should move those by the lower part of the legs avoiding contact with the sterile drapes. It must be done gently and smoothly. It is essential that the Mayo tray is free of the patient's legs.

Draping

The nurse must be available at this stage also in case her help is required to hold a limb or move some piece of apparatus. She must receive the tray after the skin cleaning is completed.

Preparation of the Basin Stand

The basin wrapped in two pack covers is already in position in the stand. The circulating nurse opens the outer wrap allowing the cover to drape over the stand. It is now the turn of the scrub nurse to open the inner cover. The floor nurse now prepares the bottle of sterile water for use. If it has a vacuum cap the vacuum is released in most cases by hitting the cap firmly. The cap is then removed and the water is poured into the basin. There should be a clear line of safety between the basin and the bottle. The bottle should always be held at an angle so that no drops can fall from the side of the bottle into the sterile basin. The cap should not be returned to the bottle or the water left to be used at a later date.

The Theatre

The theatre should be kept tidy during the operation. The circulating nurse must be prepared to help any member of the team to see to this.

Aseptic Technique

It is possible for the nurse to view the sterile field from a distance. She may detect any break in the aseptic technique and be able to report it immediately.

Messages in Theatre

If a message has to be relayed to a member of the operating team the nurse must decide first whether it is urgent enough or whether it cannot wait until the end of the operation. If this is so she will inform the scrub nurse who will in turn tell the person involved at the most convenient time.

It is not advisable to interrupt the surgeon directly.

The nurse must of course be sure to give the message at the end of the operation if she has decided that it was not sufficiently urgent at the time.

Mopping of the Forehead

The circulating nurse should be aware of any perspiration on the forehead of any member of the operating team. She should be ready with a small moist sponge to remove the perspiration before the dangerous stage of it fouling the wound is reached.

A swab must not be used as this will interfere with the swab count.

Care should be taken that there is no contamination.

Pouring Lotions

The receptable must be brought to the edge of the trolley or held by the scrub nurse before the circulating nurse begins to pour into it (holding the label on the bottle uppermost).

She should never lean over the sterile field to carry out this duty.

The solution to be poured will of course have been checked, the label shown to the scrub nurse, and the lotion named audibly.

Aerosol Sprays

Sometimes the nurse is asked to spray into the wound. She must follow the instructions on the container e.g. she may have to shake the container.

Standing well back from and above the sterile field the contents are sprayed into the wound in the precise direction instructed by the surgeon or sister.

Cleaning Spectacles

This is frequently a request. Great care is required in removing and replacing them.

Drainage Equipment

The necessary apparatus should be ready for the moment it is required e.g. chest drainage apparatus.

The End of the Operation

After the patient has left the theatre the nurse will untie all the operating team. All equipment used for this operation is cleared away and the theatre is prepared for the next operation.

30
What Kind of Catheters are used in Surgery?

Depezzer Catheter

This catheter is used to drain a cavity. Sometimes used for chest drainage.

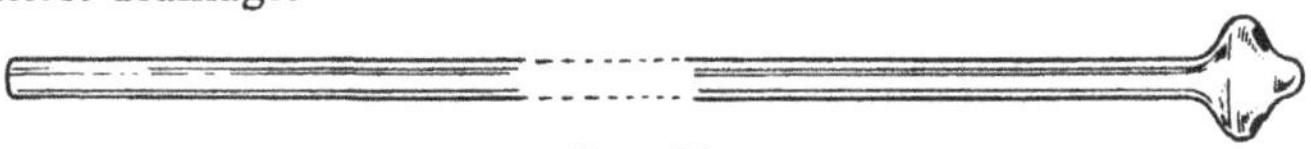

Fig. 36

Balloon Catheter

This is a self-retaining catheter. It is most commonly inserted into the bladder. The balloon is filled with water.

Fig. 37

Whistle-tip Catheter

This catheter is frequently used by the anaesthetist for endotrachael suction. It may also be used for drainage.

Fig. 38

Jacques Catheter

This catheter is very commonly used and suitable for general use.

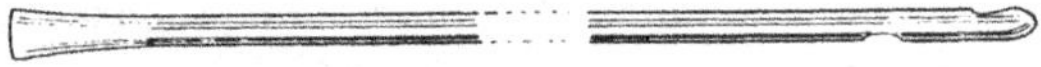

Fig. 39

Ureteric Catheter

These are passed through a cystoscope prior to retrograde pyelography. The right and left are identified by different colours.

Oseophageal Tube

This is inserted pre-operatively in many gastric operations.

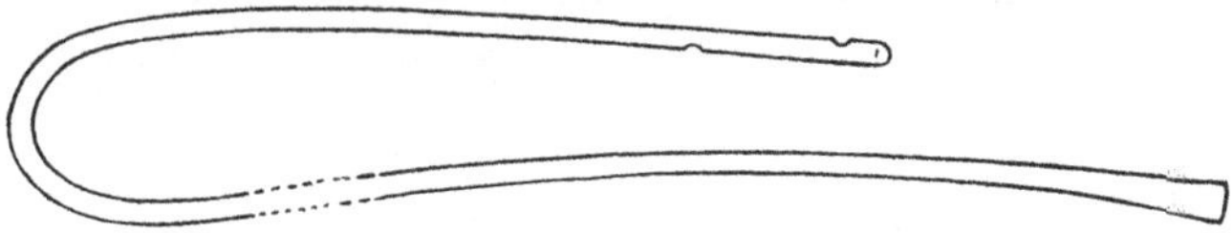

Fig. 40

Levine Tube

This is used in gastric and bowel surgery for gastric irrigation.

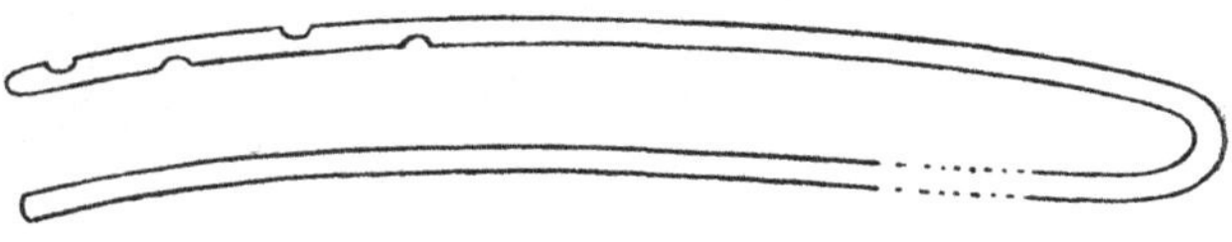

Fig. 41

Sengstaten Tube

This may be used for arresting the bleeding in oesophageal varices. It consists of an inflatable bag.

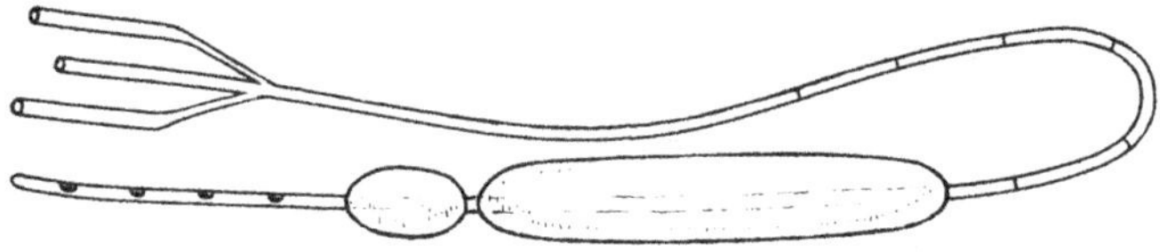

Fig. 42

31

How does the Nurse care for and know the Instruments in the Theatre?

Instruments vary in structure and design to meet a particular purpose. Surgeons do have individual preferences. The nurse must remember that a craftsman requires his own tools.

Care of the Instruments

Many instruments have delicate parts to them and warrant great respect and dare in the handling of them.

1 Instruments must be inspected before and after use in case there are any imperfections e.g. a piece missing. It must also be noted whether the instrument is bent or damaged in any way.
2 Instruments should be tested to make sure they are in good working order. Any instrument not passing this inspection should be laid aside for repair and attention.
3 Instruments must not be used for any other purpose than for that for which they have been designed.

4 Proper use will keep instruments in good order.
5 Lensed instruments must be handled carefully and protection be provided for them by the container.
6 Special racks are used to hold fine instruments in place.
7 The cleaning of instruments must be carefully carried out. Ultra-sonic cleaning machines may be used.
8 Protection from breakage and distortion must be provided.
9 The use of cleaning agents must be supervised in case of abrasion to any fine instrument or lensed instrument.
10 Instruments consisting of both metal and glass should not be autoclaved because of the unequal expansion of each material on heating.
11 Manufacturer's instructions on the care of any new instruments must be strictly adhered to.
12 Instruments should be rinsed through as soon as possible after use. This prevents tissue crusting or blood clotting inside a part of the instrument.

32

What are the Various Instruments used in the Theatre?

Dissection

In most operations it is necessary to cut through the skin and then into the deeper tissue. The separation of the tissues is called dissection. This may be blunt dissection or sharp dissection depending on the instrument used.

Retraction

The surgeon requires to have ready access to the region

for operation so retraction is required to pull aside any structures which prevent this access.

The whole process is called the Surgical Approach.

The Knife

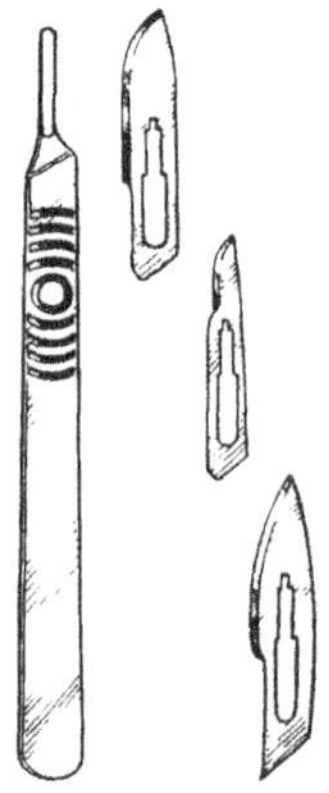

Fig. 43 Bard Parker Handle and Blades

The knife is the main cutting instrument. It has many variations. In most cases there is a handle with a disposable blade. There are a great many varieties of the shapes of blades. There are a few different sizes of handles depending on the purpose for which the knife is required.

Amputation Knife

This may still be used but a dissection and isolation of large vessels does not necessitate its use so frequently. Great care must be taken by the nurse when she is packing and and handling this knife.

Tenotomy Knife

This is a sharp pointed knife designed to make a small incision in the skin and to cut through fascia or tendon. This knife is used in orthopaedic and plastic surgery.

Nasal Septal Knife

This is a swivel knife used in nasal surgery.

Myringotome

This is a smaller triangular knife with a long fine handle. It is used to make an incision in the ear drum to allow the release of pus or serum.

Eye Knife or Scleratome

There are a few variations of this knife but all are very fine and very easily damaged if they are not well protected.

Meniscectomy Knives

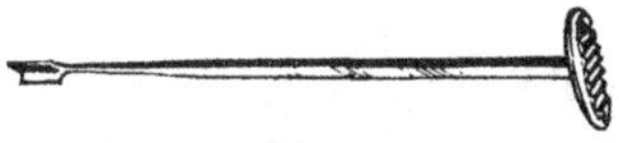

Fig. 44

These are usually in sets of three and are used to cut the cartilage of the knee.

Diathermy Point

This is often used to cut muscle.

Scissors

The types of scissors can be divided broadly into the following categories:-

Dissection Scissors

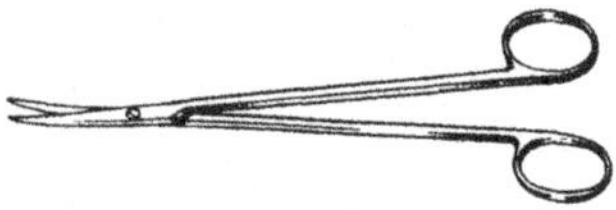

Fig. 45

These may be short, long, and extra long depending on the area of surgery. They should never be used for cutting sutures.

Eye Scissors

These can be sharp-pointed or blunt-pointed and have short handles. As well as being used for eye surgery they are used for fine dissecting e.g. vascular work.

Mayo Scissors

They are used to cut muscle, sutures, and any other tissue that is not so delicate.

Suture Scissors

The scrub nurse should always keep an identifiable pair of scissors on her trolley especially for use for all the various purposes for which she may require them.

Wire Cutting Scissors

These scissors are a special pair used for cutting wire. A heavy pair of Mayo scissors can be used for cutting wire as long as they are kept specifically for the purpose.

Tonsil Scissors

These are long scissors with a curve on the shaft and have sharp points.

Artery Forceps

The artery forcep is used to occlude a blood vessel. A tie is placed around and tied as the forcep is released so that the knot is completed.

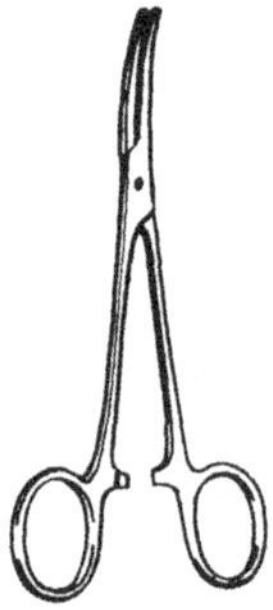

Fig. 46

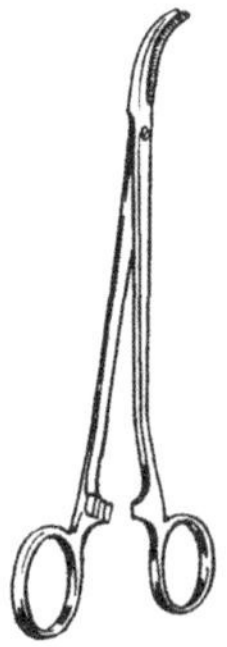

Fig. 47

Artery forceps are also many and varied. They have a screw or a box joint—the latter being longer lasting.

Artery forceps can be short, medium, long, and extra long; straight, curved, or angled; with sharp, blunt, or fine points.

Mosquito Forceps

These are small fine forceps for fine delicate work.

Diathermy Forceps

Those are attached to the diathermy machine lead and used to co-agulate blood vessels.

Dissecting Forceps

They are used to allow the surgeon to hold tissue accurately. Again there are many types. Each surgeon has a preferance for dissecting forceps according to his personal custom.

They are supplied fine, heavy, non-toothed, toothed, long, and short. Each one has its own particular purpose e.g. one is especially designed to hold lung tissue.

The teeth of dissecting forceps should be well protected and always thoroughly examined after use.

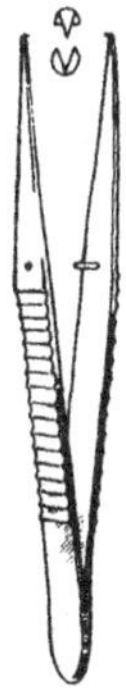

Fig. 48

Dissectors

These are flat blunt instruments used for blunt dissection. Sometimes a hole is present so that a ligature can be passed through the instrument and then under the vessel e.g. a McDonald's dissector.

Towel Clips

Towel clips have sharp points or blunt ends. They are used to hold towels and drapes in place. Diathermy and suction may also be held in position by another variety of clip.

Care must be taken with the sharp points both in handling them and in preventing damage to the drapes.

Tissue Forceps

These are used to hold tissue either as retractors or while dissecting is taking place. Some are heavy and are used on tough tissue. (e.g. Lane's Forceps). Others are fine e.g. Babcock's which are non-traumatic.

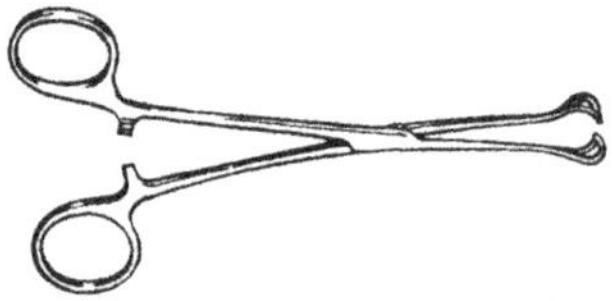

Fig. 49

Retractors

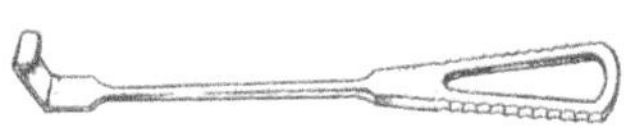

Fig. 50

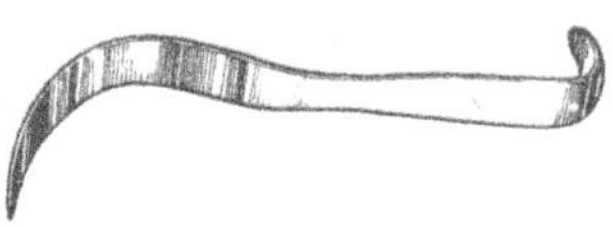

Fig. 51

These are many and varied. They can usually be divided into sizes.

1 Small

Used in fine and superficial surgery. They are supplied either single hook or double hook.

2 Medium

e.g. Langenbeck's retractors which are used for minor surgery such as herniorrhaphy and appendicectomy. The rake type can also be used in these circumstances.

3 Large

This includes all abdominal retractors e.g. Deaver's and Morris retractors.

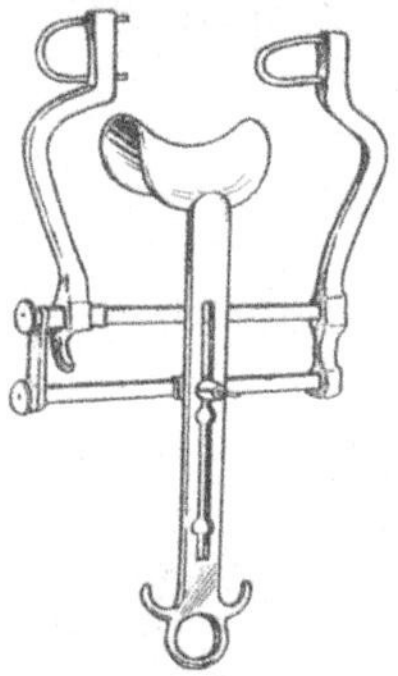

Fig. 52

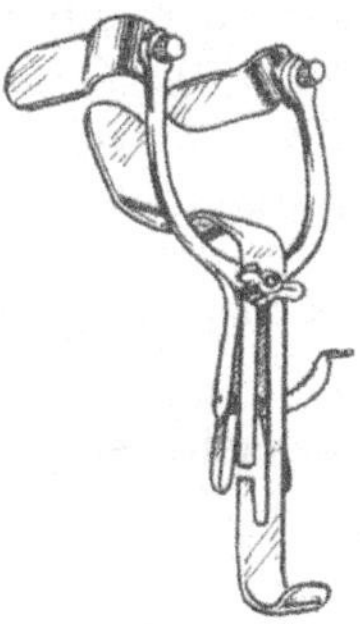

Fig. 53

Other types are malleable, illuminated, self-retaining, etc. Some self-retaining types have detachable blades so that different widths and lengths can be used, according to the size of the wound and the size of the patient. (Figs. 52, 53).

Needle Holders

Again these are many varieties—long, short, fine, heavy, etc. A needle holder is one of the instruments a surgeon becomes attached to and accustomed to.

A newer type of needle holder has a diamond jaw. This prevents the grip from becoming worn. Some others have ratchets.

Chisels and Osteotomes

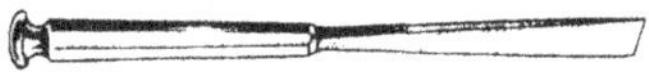

Fig. 54

This is sometimes difficult for the theatre nurse to identify. The chisel has a flat surface.

Bone Instruments

There are many instruments all with their own particular use:-

bone-holding forceps, drills, saws, gouges.

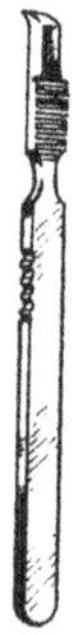

Fig. 55 Periosteal Elevator

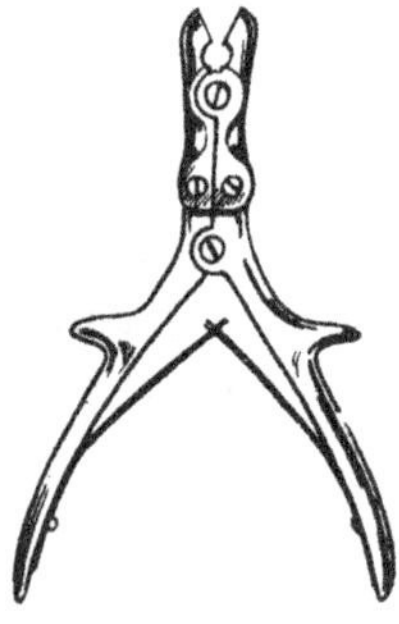

Fig. 57 Bone Nibbling Forceps

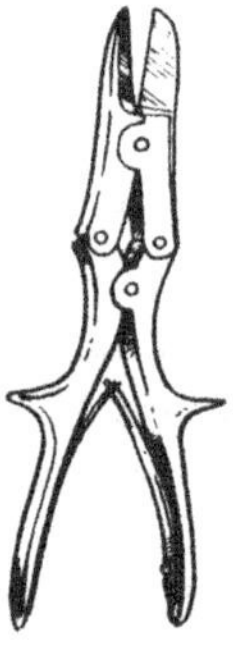

Fig. 56 Bone Cutting Forceps

Accessory Instruments

Those are devices to apply to other instruments. They will include mallets, screw drivers, suction nozzles, etc.

Bowel Clamps

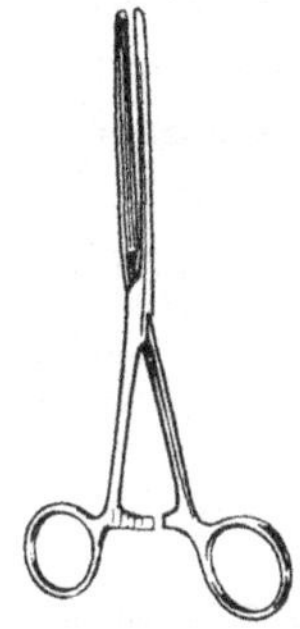

Fig. 58

There are many types of these. Some are twin-locking used for anastomosis. Basically there are two main types:-

1 The occlusion clamp which is placed on the part to be anastomosed together e.g. Doyen's.
2 The crushing clamp which is being placed on the part being removed e.g. Peyr's.

It is essential that the theatre nurse can apply her knowledge of anatomy and physiology to enable her to select the correct instrument. The smaller finer instrument will be used for paediatric, opthalmic, aural, vascular, brain, nurse, and facial surgeries.

The Theatre Nurse must know the use of and the care of every Instrument. The special names can be discovered as her experience increases.

33
What are the Various Endoscopes?

Laryngoscope (Fig. 5, page 35)

This is an instrument used to examine the larynx. It is used by the anaesthetist mainly to insert endotracheal tubes.

Bronchoscope

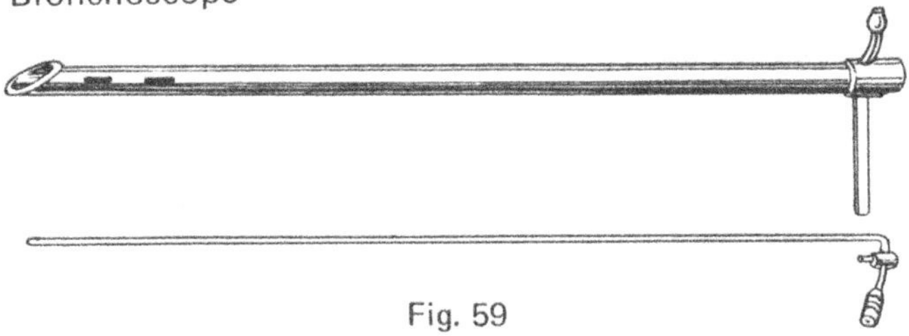

Fig. 59

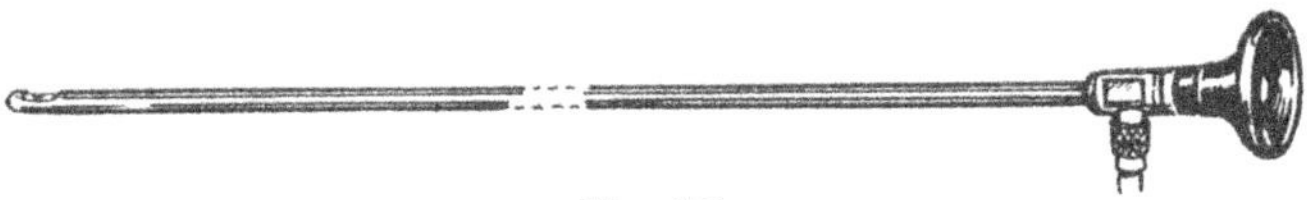

Fig. 60

This is an instrument used to examine the bronchi. A biopsy may also be taken when bronchoscopy is performed.

Oesophagoscope

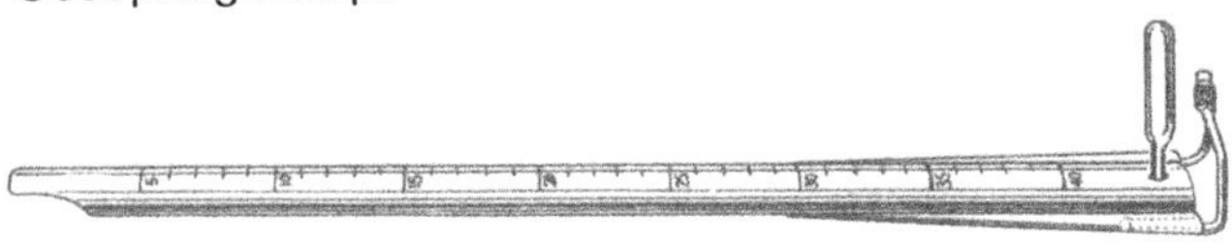

Fig. 61

This is an instrument used to examine the oesophagus. Oesophagoscopy is frequently performed to obtain a biopsy or remove a foreign body.

Gastroscope

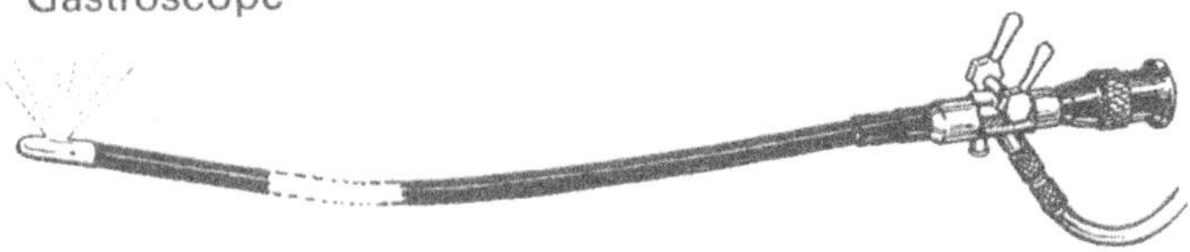

Fig. 62

This is a flexible instrument used to examine the stomach.

Sigmoidoscope

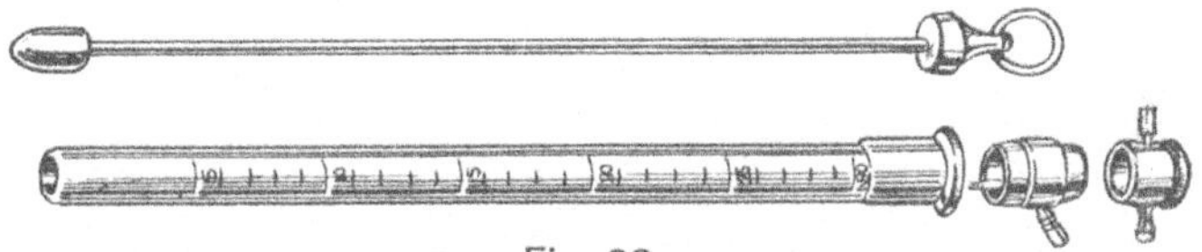

Fig. 63

This is an instrument used to examine the sigmoid colon. A biopsy is usually taken at sigmoidoscopy.

Proctoscope

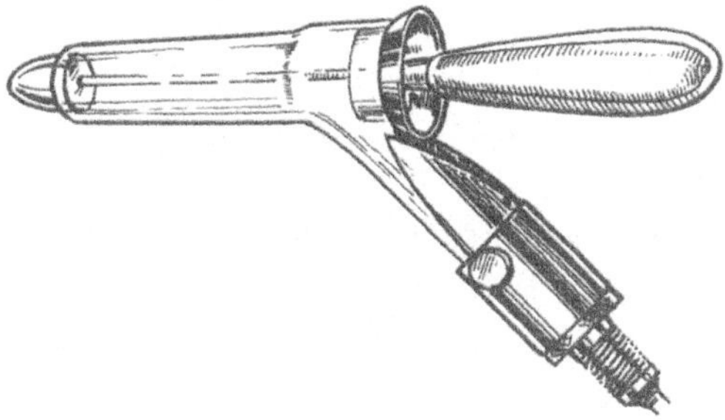

Fig. 64

This is an instrument used to examine the rectum.

Cystoscope

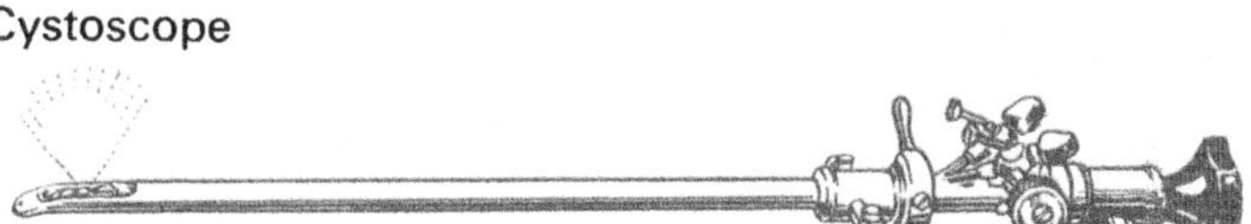

Fig. 65

This is an instrument used to examine the bladder. Biopsy may be undertaken and ureteric catheters may be inserted on cystoscopic examination. There is a large range of types of cystoscopes.

Laparoscope

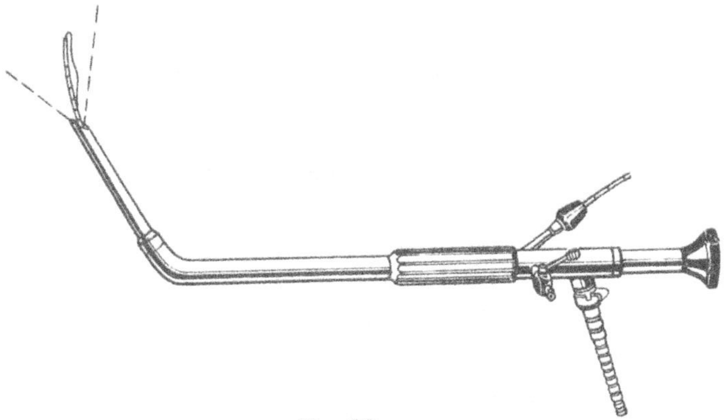

Fig. 66

This is an instrument used to examine the contents of the female pelvis.

Choledochoscope

This is an instrument used to examine the common bile duct. Provision is made for irrigation.

34

What are Some of the Drains used in Surgery?

Fluid or air may be drained away in a variety of ways. The particular type of drain is put into the area from which the fluid or air would be likely to pass. They are usually brought out to the surface through a stab wound in the skin away from the main incision. Types include:-

1 Rubber Tube

The rubber tube can be of varying thicknesses and lengths. It should be soft but firm. If the walls of the tubing collapse then the fluid will not drain.

The tip of a piece of rubber tubing approximately 6-8 inches (18cm.) long is cut with a bevel as are a few holes below the tip.

The scrub nurse must cut and check the holes carefully before handing the tube to the surgeon in case a loose fragment of tubing could become dislodged.

This rubber tube drain is a fairly common form of drainage and is used in general surgery to drain the cavity or space around an organ. e.g. cholecystectomy.

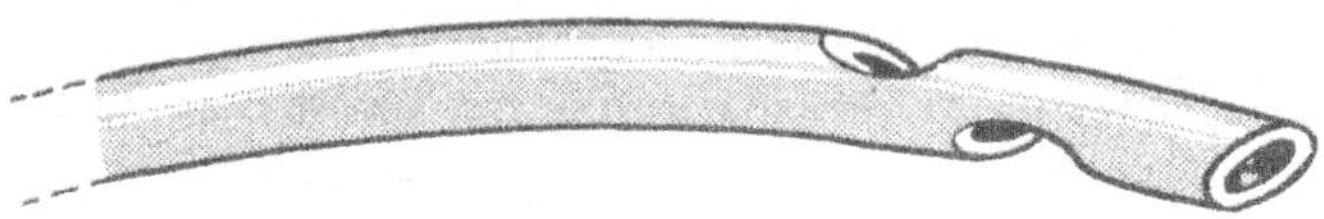

Fig. 67

2 Penrose or Cigarette Drain

This is a fine latex rubber tube with a strip of gauze pulled through the lumen serving as a wick. There are various widths of this drain. Very often it is used as a fine sub-cutaneous drain e.g. after thyroidectomy.

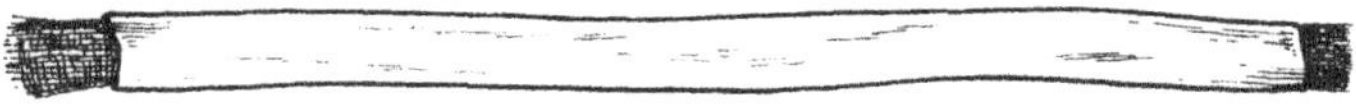

Fig. 68

3 Corrugated Rubber Drain

This is as its name suggests a series of corrugations and gutters. The surgeon will select the length and width. The end is usually tapered before insertion.

This drain is commonly used in surgery in a variety of situations.

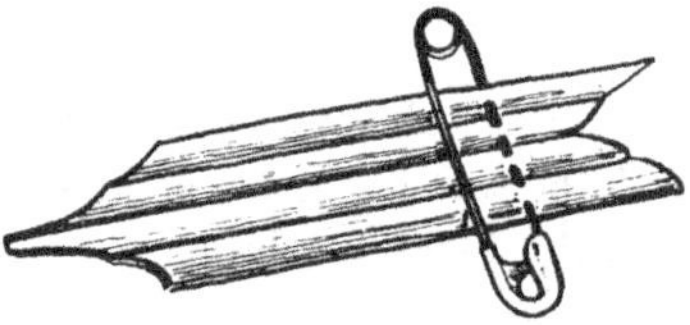

Fig. 69

4 T-Tube

This tube can be made of rubber, latex rubber, or nylon. It is used after the common bile duct has been explored.

The ends are bevelled and cut to fit the common bile duct.

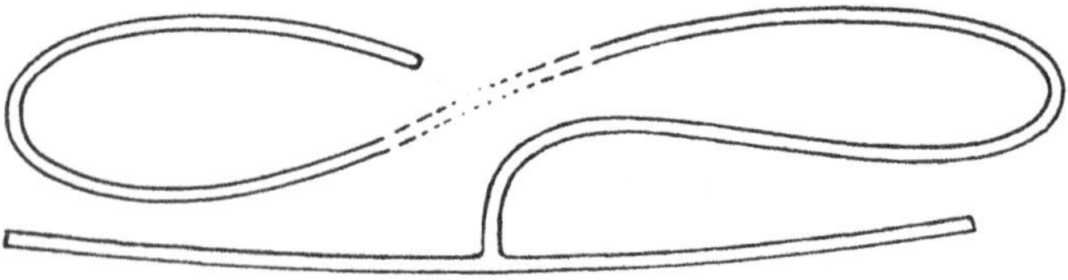

Fig. 70

Catheters

A catheter can be used for spontaneous drainage or be indwelling. The catheter may be connected up to suction for continuous drainage.

Some catheters are self-retaining e.g. they have an inflatable balloon at the tip which is filled by fluid to keep the catheter in situ.

Others are anchored in position by a catgut stitch.

Chest Drain

This type of drainage must be completely understood by theatre nurses. One or two drainage tubes or catheters can be used to drain the chest. The apparatus consists of a sterile bottle with a known quantity of sterile water. The bottle is fitted with a bung in which are inserted two tubes–one long extending below the water level, the other short. The tube or catheter from the patient's chest is connected by a longer piece of tubing to the longer glass tube in the bottle. It is imperative that the bottle always remains below the level of the patient thus preventing re-entrance and therefore the loss of negative pressure of fluid into the chest cavity.

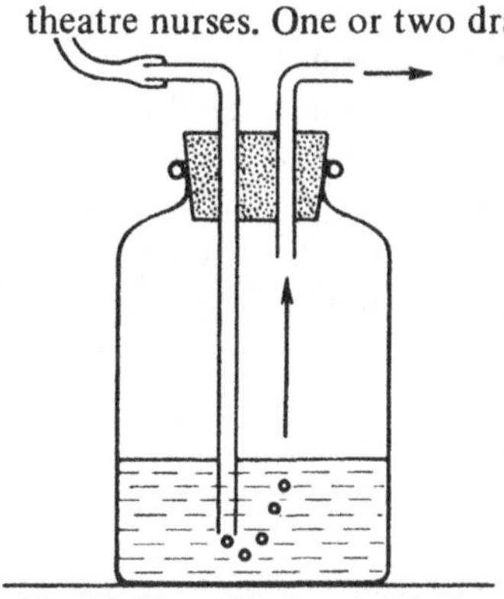

Fig.71 Chest Drainage Bottle

Two large clamps should always be available in case it is

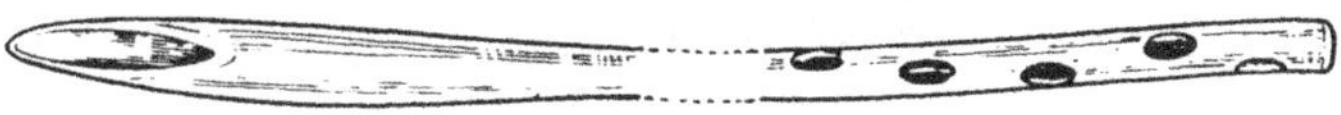

Fig. 72 Chest Drainage Tube

necessary to seal the tubing e.g. when changing the bottle or turning the patient.

Vacuum Drain

This aids wound healing by a method of closed suction. It is used in operations where there are no complications anticipated. A needle attached to tubing is guided through the tissue from the site to be drained and brought out to the skin. The drainage tube is then connected to the vacuum bottle.

General Remarks

An adequate selection of sizes and variations of catheters and drain should always be available at the time of surgery.

Appropriate connections, clamps, and additional lengths of tubing should always be to hand.

Unfortunately it is not always possible for the surgeon to predict exactly for the theatre nurse the nature of the drain that he will require. A large selection must be available in the theatre area.

A large variety of connections are also necessary if the drain is to be connected to tubing or drainage bottle.

It is absolutely essential that the presence of a drain in the wound is reported to the Ward Staff when the Patient returns there from Theatre.

35

What are the Various Dressings Applied in the Theatre?

The good circulating nurse always has the dressing materials ready before the end of the operation. Familiarity with the practice and preferences of each surgeon is essential.

The tendency these days with clean wounds is to have a very light dressing or in some cases a sealing spray and no dressing.

The type of adhesive tape used these days is also light and non-traumatic.

Thought must be given to the purpose of the dressing, the size of the patient, and the mobility required of the patient after the operation.

The Purpose of a Dressing

1 to eliminate all bacteria from the incision area.
2 to protect the wound from injury.
3 to keep down swelling.
4 to absorb drainage.
5 to immobilise an area.
6 to give support to the area e.g. after a skin graft.
7 to make the patient more comfortable.

However there are certain common operations requiring special dressing routines:-

Colostomy Dressing

Tulle Gras is placed around the colostomy. Swabs may be cut to fit over the piece of bowel.

Haemorrhoidectomy Dressing

Tulle Gras is placed around the drain. Swabs are applied also and plenty of wool and a T-bandage.

Mastectomy Dressing

This requires swabs, cotton wool padding, and a crepe bandage firmly applied.

Varicose Vein Dressing

After stripping of the vein swabs, gamgee, or wool are applied to the incision sites. The leg is then firmly bandaged with crepe bandage.

Ear Dressing

Swabs and a light type of bandage e.g. Kling are applied around the head.

Tracheostomy Dressing

Sometimes a butterfly dressing is prepared and placed around the tube. Alternatively tulle gras can be used. This procedure does vary according to the post-operative treatment of the patient.

Knee Dressing

This dressing has swabs, many layers of wool, and a crepe bandage.

Another layer of wool and another crepe bandage may also be applied.

Plaster of Paris Bandage

It is important that the theatre nurse leaves the patient's skin completely clean before applying this bandage. If there is any oozing of blood sufficient padding should be applied first.

Plaster wool is then bandaged on.

A bucket of water is required. The temperature of this water depends on the type of plaster being used. The main rule is to follow the manufacturer's instructions in the matter of the temperature of the water.

After application of the plaster of Paris the skin must be well cleaned by the nurse. If this is not done it can be very uncomfortable later on.

Dressing Several Wounds

If there is more than one wound to be dressed each is dealt with separately. Very often a drain is lead out through a stab wound. This would is dressed with plenty of swabs and wool.

The main incision will be sealed off by using waterproof adhesive thus preventing any contamination from the exudate from the drain.

There are many aids to dressing wounds available. Gauze bandages are almost completely replaced by tube gauze and Netelast.

Practice in the use of the applicators of tube gauge etc. is required by the circulating nurse.

Some surgeons prefer to apply the dressings themselves.

In this case the nurse should have all the equipment needed at hand and be ready with a helping hand if asked.

36

What are the Various Kinds of Suture Material?

There are two main types of suture material:-

1 Absorbable

This is digested and absorbed by the tissues during the process of wound healing.

2 Non-Absorbable

The tissues will not absorb these sutures. They remain in the tissues permanently except when removed surgically e.g. skin suture.

Absorbable Sutures

1 Catgut

This is the most commonly used absorbable suture material. The word is said to be derived from the Arabic word 'kit' meaning a fiddle.

Catgut comes from sheep intestines and passes through many processing stages before being finally presented in its sterile state. Sterilisation is by gamma-radiation. There are two kinds:-

Plain Catgut

This is untreated after processing. The absorption rate of this is influenced by many factors such as the kind of tissue, the physical condition of the patient, or the presence of infection. Plain catgut is used in tissue that will heal quickly. It will be absorbed in five to ten days.

Chromic Catgut

This material is just plain catgut immersed in a chromium salt solution.

There can be different degrees of this chromacizing process, e.g. medium chromic, chromic, and hard. This catgut enables the wound with slow healing power to gather sufficient strength of its own before the suture is entirely absorbed.

Catgut Sizing

Scaled from large–4, 3, 2, 1, 0, 2/0, 3/0, 4/0, 5/0, 6/0, 7/0, to small.

Presentation

More usually catgut is presented in a foil or plastic

packet. Very occasionally it is supplied in a glass tube.

This packet or tube can contain a fluid which provides the catgut with maximum pliability.

The catgut should be used as soon as possible after removing it from the packet.

Catgut should be handled as little as possible as fraying will result. A gloved hand should never be drawn down the length of the catgut.

2 Fascia Lata

This is not truly absorbable but does become part of the tissue.

It is used to provide support to weakened fascial layers.

It is obtained from beef cattle and is prepared in strips in a sterile pack.

It can also be obtained from the patient's thigh and used for hernial repair.

3 Ribbon Gut

This is obtained also from cattle and may be used as a sling e.g. a kidney operation.

4 Kangaroo Tendon

This is obtained as its name suggests from the kangaroo. It is rarely used nowadays. It is a very strong suture and may be used for suturing patellar fragments.

5 Bone Wax

This is not strictly a suture. It is rubbed on the surface of the bone to arrest bleeding.

It is also presented in a pack which requires a few seconds immersion in warm sterile water.

This will soften the wax and make it pliable for the surgeon's use.

Non-Absorbable Sutures

1 Silk

Surgical silk sutures are processed from raw silk. It is widely used in a twisted or braided form.

All silk is treated with a silicone process to make it serum-proof. i.e. able to withstand the action of body fluids.

Presentation

It is presented in the same way as catgut in pre-cut lengths and attached to needles. The same sizing scale is applied to silk as to the catgut sutures.

The packet does not normally contain any fluid.

Silk is only used on tissues which are not infected or are not liable for infection.

2 Cotton

This is not as strong as silk and is not widely used.

3 Linen

This is similar to and treated in the same way as silk.

4 Human Hair

This is very fine suturing material and may be used for nerve repair.

5 Nylon

This is a synthetic material. It is available in two forms:-

multifilament
monofilament

It is very strong but because of its smooth surface the surgeon will tie three knots in contrast to two for the other materials.

6 Dacron

This is a synthetic polyester fibre. This is a strong braided suture inert in the tissues.

A size less than normal may be indicated.

It is widely used in cardio-vascular procedures.

7 Linear Polythene

This is also a synthetic material. It has a high degree of pliability and therefore easy to handle. It is used widely in plastic surgery because of minimal tissue reaction.

8 Nylon and Dacron Tape

Those tapes are available in sterile packs and are used for occlusion of vessels and for traction of fine structures.

9 Stainless Steel Wire

This is a metal suturing material.

It is presented in monostrand and multistrand sutures.

Stainless steel does not corrode and does not cause pain. It can be used when infection is present and for secondary repair.

Care should be taken when tying wire that the suture is cut close to the knot and the ends turned into the tissue.

Special wire cutters or scissors are kept for this purpose alone and should be used.

10 Silver Wire

This is similar to stainless steel but presented only in monofilament form. It is not widely used.

11 Stainless Steel Mesh and Nylon Mesh

This fine wire mesh is used widely in herniorraphy operations. The tissue is allowed to grow through the mesh strengthening the surrounding tissue. It is usually secured with silk suture.

12 Clips

Skin clips are not so widely used nowadays. The most common are Michel or Kifa which are used on the skin edges.

Other stainless steel varieties are used in neurosurgical operations to control bleeding.

37
How are the Wounds Stitched?

As women use a variety of stitches in making a dress or in embroidering a teacloth so surgeons use a variety of sutures to stitch up the wounds.

The surgeon with his experience, choice of material, and type of tissue evolves a definite suturing pattern.

The theatre nurse learns how to handle these sutures, how to hand them to the surgeon, whether the suture should be long or short, whether it should be mounted on a needle holder or for use in the surgeon's hand.

Terms

Terms can vary a great deal but with frequency of use soon become familiar.

A Suture

A suture is a piece of suture material threaded on to a needle e.g. a skin suture holds the edges of the wound together.

There are many types of suture. Here are a few:-

1 A Continuous Suture

This is a long suture where only the first and last stitches are tied.

The peritoneum is usually stitched with a continuous suture.

2 An Interrupted Suture

This can be done with a series of short pieces of suture material threaded on to needles or using atraumatic needles (i.e. needles swaged on to suture material).

Each stitch is self contained and is tied separately.

There are various methods of interrupted sutures according to the purpose the surgeon wishes to achieve.

3 A Purse String Suture

As its name suggests this is a continuous suture placed around an opening and the ends are drawn together. This is commonly used around the caecum, the appendix stump being invaginated before tying and cutting of the suture.

It is also used when a tube is inserted e.g. gastrostomy tube.

4 A Tension Suture

This suture is interrupted and usually of stronger suture material. Quite often a piece of rubber tubing is threaded through thus preventing the suture cutting the skin.

It is used to relieve strain on the wound suture line in obese patients and for infected wounds.

5 A Stay Suture

A pair of stay sutures are often used. The sutures are inserted into the structure e.g. the common bile duct.

The needle is removed, the ends brought together, and forceps are applied.

The surgeon's assistant will hold the two sutures taut to enable the operator to cut into the structure.

6 An Anchoring Suture

This can be used to anchor a drainage tube to the skin. A non-absorbable suture will be used.

It can also be used to hold a drainage tube inside a cavity e.g. a T-Tube in a common bile duct. An absorbable suture will be used for easy removal.

7 A Ligature

A ligature is a length of suture material used to encircle a vessel or close off a structure.

An artery forceps having been applied to the lumen of the vessel is held up by the assistant while the surgeon applies the ligature.

After the first tie the forceps are removed.

The tying is completed and the ends are cut off above the knot.

8 A Transfixion Suture

This is a length of suture material threaded on to a needle. It is applied to prevent the ligature slipping off the end of the vessel or structure e.g. transfixion of hernial sac, or the transfixion of a cystic artery.

Quite often vessels in deep tissues are dealt with in this way.

9 A Mounted Ligature

This is made using an aneurysm needle or artery forcep.

When the vessel or structure cannot be reached easily to apply the ligature then the ligature is placed on a long artery forcep and threaded into the open jaws of the artery forceps under the vessel. This is done in pairs and the ligatures should be of sufficient length for the purpose.

10 Traction Suture

This is similar to a stay suture. It is used to retract a piece of tissue or a structure e.g. the tongue during a mouth operation.

38

What Type of Needles are Used?

There are so many types of needles that mention can only be made here of a few of the more widely used ones.

A surgical needle should be identified by three parts:-

1 the eye
2 the shaft
3 the point

Needles with an Eye

NEEDLE EYES

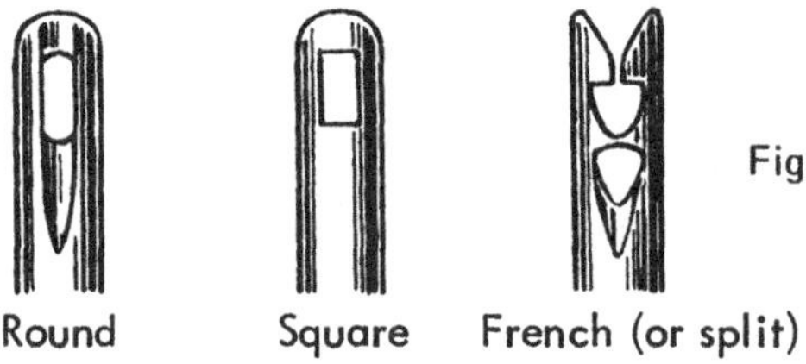

Fig. 73

These needles may be used more than once but of course must be examined after use for damage and to inspect the sharpness.

Very fine needles should be discarded after using once.

The eye of the needle may be round, square, or be of the split-eye variety. Split-eye needles can be threaded by drawing the thread over the end of the needle. A tiny spring allows the thread to pass into the eye.

To thread a needle with a round or square eye the suture material should be held between the thumb and forefinger of the left hand. Place the eye over the material as the fingers open up.

The threaded needle should show the short length i.e. one third of the whole length of the suture material.

The Shaft of the Needle

NEEDLE SHAFTS

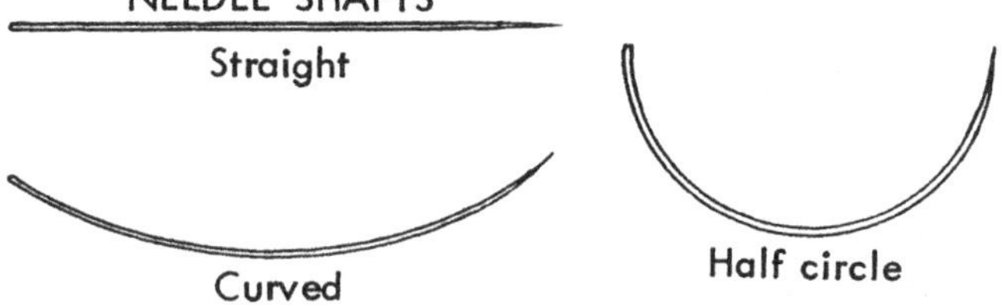

Fig. 74

The most common shapes are straight, curved, or half-circle—but many other varied shapes are available.

The Point of the Needle

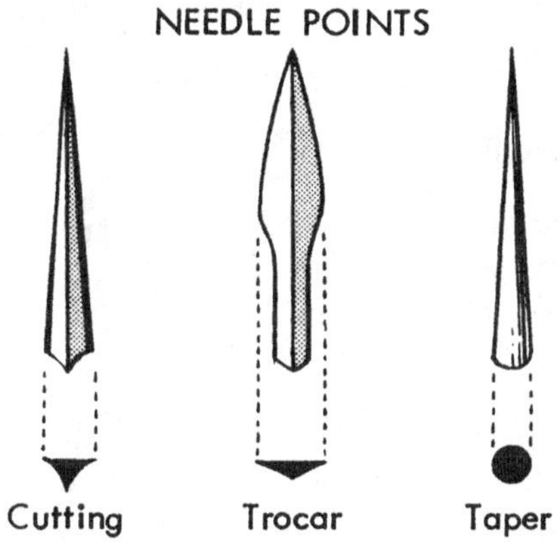

Fig. 75

The point of the surgical needle can be triangular, taper pointed, or trocar. It is important that the theatre nurse gradually learns to recognise the various types of needle used in her particular place of work.

Atraumatic Sutures

Additional advantages of the atraumatic suture are that no threading is required and that a new sharp needle is provided for each use.

Atraumatic sutures come to the theatre ready for use already sterilised.

Atraumatic sutures are presented with either a single needle or in the case of a double-ended suture two needles—one at either end.

Fortunately for the theatre nurse most of the needles used in surgery now are atraumatic. They are so called because the needle is swaged on to the suture material in a uniform combination.

A strand threaded through a needle eye will cause more trauma as two thicknesses of that strand will have to pass through the tissues.

Presenting the Needle

When using a needle holder the needle should be gripped about one third of the way along the needle shaft from the eye end, and grasped only at the tip of the needle holder.

A flattened portion is found on the shaft of the atraumatic needle.

Straight needles and large needles do not need to be mounted on a needle holder. The surgeon holds them in his hand for suturing.

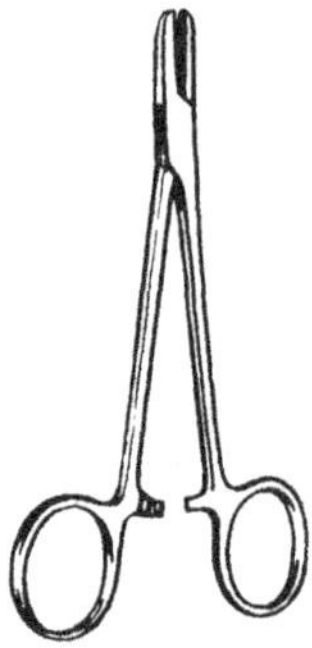

Fig. 76 Stitch Holder

The Size of the Needle

The size of the needle is obviously determined by the type of tissues. Obviously fine needles and fine suture material will be required for delicate tissue.

The size of the wound and the position that the surgeon is operating also determines the size of the needle e.g. to suture a vessel deep down in the abdominal cavity the surgeon will require a small, half circle fine needle and thread on a needle holder.

All theatre nurses find the understanding of sutures a little confusing at first. It is only with experience as the circulating nurse and the scrub nurse that the subject suddenly falls into place.

Atraumatic needles should be identified by the needle

and the suture material and not by the code number of the suture firm.

39

What is the Procedure for Dealing with an Infected Operation?

Sometimes it is known beforehand that a patient's wound is infected or that the patient has a known infection. If this is so then the operation is placed later on the list.

In some operating suites a separate room is kept available for such infected cases where their surgery is performed.

Nursing Procedure Before the Operation

The room is cleared of all unnecessary furniture and equipment.

The trolley is prepared with the necessary instruments, dressings, lotions, sutures, and accessories.

As many disposable items as possible are used.

The nurse must anticipate well to avoid any traffic in and out of the theatre once the operation has begun.

The minimum of staff are selected to be at the operation.

Disposable bags for the reception of linen and soiled material are made ready.

No equipment should be removed from the theatre until after the operation is over.

Nursing Procedure After the Operation

The surgeon is asked to place his gowns straight into the linen disposal bag. All other linen is placed in the same bag.

All dressings and other disposable materials—including gloves—are deposited into the appropriate bag.

The instruments are placed in a receptacle containing a strong antiseptic solution and left for a definite period in it.

They can then be rinsed and autoclaved before thorough cleaning.

Alternatively the instruments can be thoroughly scrubbed and washed prior to tray-setting and re-autoclaving.

The choice of routine depends on the facilities in the theatre.

All furniture used is washed thoroughly with a stronger solution of antiseptic and disposal bags are placed in another wrapping and removed from the area immediately.

Personnel must change all clothing before proceeding with another operation.

Circumstances vary so much with the layout of each theatre suite. However it is essential that whatever the routine is that is in practice in the theatre in which you work it must be carried out implicitly.

40

How does the Scrub Nurse prepare herself?

Appearance

The scrub nurse should see that her dress sleeves are well above her elbows and that the belt of her dress cannot contaminate anything i.e. tied at the back or side.

The mask she is wearing should be tied securely and comfortably.

Her finger nails should be short and clean.

Her hands and arms should be free from any abrasions or septic spots.

The Surgical Scrub

The basic principle is to remove bacteria from the skin.

It is not possible to make the hands sterile and because of this the hands and arms must not come into contact with the outside of either the gown or the gloves.

Procedure

The water should be adjusted to a suitable temperature and the arms and hands held under the taps.

An antiseptic scrub lotion e.g. Phisohex or Betadine is applied to the hands from a container usually operated from a foot pedal.

Rinsing takes place after this preliminary wash.

After this stage the hands should always be held higher than the elbows.

A sterilised nail brush is now used to clean the nails.

After a rinse and discard of the nail brush the lotion is applied again and a full wash takes place of the arms up to the elbows and of the hands themselves. Particular attention should be paid to the spaces between the fingers.

When rinsing is taking place the water is allowed to drip from the elbows.

The whole wash should take about four minutes.

Taps are turned off with the back of the arm or by the circulating nurse.

Drying of the Hands

A sterile towel is obtained (particularly avoiding dripping on to any part of the sterile field). The towel should be opened out full length. Care should be taken that it does not touch the front of the theatre dress.

The arms and hands are dried in such a way that a clean and dry part of the towel is used for each part.

The towel is discarded after this.

Powdering

If powder or cream is used then the powder packet is opened and the powder is poured on to the hands. This procedure should also be carried out away from the sterile field.

Gowning

The following is the general method although there are local individual differences in this procedure.

1 A sterile gown is picked up, unrolled, and opened.
2 The two arms are inserted at the same time.(Sterile gowns are folded before sterilising in such a way that the outside of the gown connot be touched by the clean hands–thus leaving a completely sterile surface).
The circulating nurse helps the scrub nurse to don the gown by putting each hand into the inner side of the gown at the shoulders and pulling it over.
4 The fastening is then made avoiding any contamination. (The circulating nurse must make herself familiar with the fastening method of the gown used–whether it has tapes, velcro fastening, or have a special back covering to manipulate).
5 The scrub nurse during this period keeps her arms extended and the elbows slightly flexed.

Gloving

Again before sterilising the gloves are packed with cuffs

turned up thus allowing the clean hands to pick up the gloves by the cuff and therefore maintaining the sterility of the outside of the glove.

The left glove is picked up by the cuff and put on.

By inserting the sterile left gloved hand under the cuff of the right hand glove this is put on.

A pleat is made in the sleeve of the gown if stockinette cuffs are not part of the gown. Then the cuffs are folded back on both gloves over this sleeve.

Removing a Gown

Again, in order to protect arms and hands from contamination from the outside of the gown and the gloves a special routine is followed.

1 The circulating nurse will unfasten the gown.
2 The gown is brought off each shoulder and removed over the arms everting the cuffs of the gloves. The arms and the gown are kept away from the body.
3 The gloves are removed by handling the everted inner cuffs only.

Practice is essential for these procedures. Soon they become automatic. Hands should never be in any other position than above the waist when nurse is wearing a sterile gown and gloves.

There are certain areas liable to contamination and therefore they are not considered sterile.

1 below the waist
2 the neckline and shoulder area
3 under the arms
4 the back of the gown

41

How does the Scrub Nurse assist the Surgeon?

The scrub nurse has certain responsibilities both to surgeon and patient:-

1 to maintain a state of asepsis
2 to anticipate as far as possible the needs of the operating team during the process of the operation
3 to be able to supply these needs
4 to carry out a meticulous swab, instrument, and needle count
5 to practice good patient care
6 to have excellent operative technique

She performs her duties after donning sterile gown, and gloves within a sterile area of the operating theatre. Here are some of the duties she will perform.

Preparing the Trolley

She lays or arranges her instrument trolley in the manner that she is to use it for the operation. It is essential that she knows the position and state of all the contents on it.

She assembles the contents ready for use with the help of her operation card.

The Mayo Tray

This small instrument tray is usually draped by the scrub nurse and laid with instruments for the surgeon to use.

When the time comes she will instruct the circulating nurse to push it carefully over the operating table.

Drapes

These should be prepared in the order in which they are to be used.

Extra drapes may be needed for a special procedure e.g. if X-rays are taken.

Swabs

After checking all the swabs in the pack she must be aware of the number allocated to the operation site and have a strict note of this throughout the operation. Dissecting swabs can be mounted on their holding forceps ready for use.

Blades

The required number and sizes are dispensed by the circulating nurse. The blades are placed on the handles carefully using an artery forceps.

In the same way the blade is removed using an artery forceps.

Blades should always be removed by the scrub nurse before she leaves her trolley for cleaning. It is essential also that she does this with a downward movement away from herself and other staff. The blade could easily break and cause injury.

It is customary to discard the blade used for the skin incision.

Sutures

The scrub nurse will have the sutures given to her by the circulating nurse. The sutures should not be opened till required.

To open the foil suture packet:-

1 the packet is torn across

2 the suture is slipped on to the finger
3 the free end is gripped and the length allowed to uncoil
4 the whole length is pulled gently—removing any kinks
5 gloved hands should not be run along the catgut as fraying will result from this
6 ligatures may be cut in lengths
7 a ligature is presented to the surgeon held at both ends and slightly taut
8 atraumatic sutures will be mounted on needle holders

The scrub nurse must always note that the needle is returned to her and it is kept for her count.

The needle holder is placed over the flattened piece of the needle and is then handed to the surgeon with the right hand. The needle is now in position ready for suturing.

The other end is handed gently over to the assistant taking care that it is not caught up in any swabs or instruments.

Scissors for cutting are then given to the assistant.

Sutures must never be allowed to dangle but must always be under the observation of the scrub nurse.

N.B. A little rethinking may need to be done about all this if the surgeon concerned happens to be left-handed!!!!

Instruments and Equipment

A constant watch is kept by the scrub nurse to ensure the working efficiency of the instruments and apparatus. The field around the incision is kept clear and tidy. Instruments are replaced into their correct position e.g. a self-retaining retractor is closed ready for use again.

Tissue and blood is removed from artery forceps.

Both the Mayo tray and instrument trolley must be kept in the original state of order.

Handling of the Instruments

This is a procedure that requires hours of practice outwith the operation.

Surgeons differ in the method they prefer the scrub nurse to hand instruments. However he generally wishes to see the instrument he is about to use.

Forceps and instruments with finger grips are held near the middle and should be placed firmly into the surgeon's hand.

If the forceps is curved the curve usually rests over the scrub nurse's hand so that the point is facing the wound when placed in the surgeon's hand.

Blades should be carefully handled. Pay particular attention that the blade if allowed to slip cannot injure either the scrub nurse or the surgeon.

The blades of self-retaining retractors must always be closed before handing them to the surgeon.

The Scrub Nurse and the Circulating Nurse must work as a team. The Scrub Nurse must be constantly one step—or maybe more ahead of the Surgeon.

Constant awareness of the operative procedure will produce a smooth-running operation.

42

How does the Theatre Nurse Care for the Patient after an Anaesthetic?

Recovery Area

The patient in most instances is transported to the recovery area where he may stay for any time up to an hour.

Sometimes the recovery ward may be some distance from the operating theatre or the patient may even have to be returned directly to the ward from which he came, via lifts and corridors.

Transfer to Trolley

The patient is transferred from the operating table to a trolley or to his own bed. Great care must be exercised by all the team that the patient is lifted gently and again that he is laid in a comfortable position.

Exposure must be avoided and the patient kept warm.

Drains and other attachments are supported and connected up if necessary.

Resuscitation Equipment

The transfer trolley should be fitted out with resuscitation equipment. This will include an oxygen supply and mask, portable suction apparatus and a catheter, and an Ambu or similar resuscitator.

The anaesthetist and surgeon will determine the position that the patient will take up on the bed or trolley.

Return of the Patient to Bed

The tonsil position is chosen for many patients returning from theatre and always for nasal and throat surgery.

The patient is placed on his side–a pillow being inserted at his back to prevent him rolling backwards:-

1 He lies slightly forward with a pillow in front and between the legs to prevent him from falling into the prone position.
2 The head will be lowered slightly.

3 The patient must also be protected from any injury such as a leg or arm slipping off the trolley.

4 It must be remembered also that he may still be insensitive to pain and his body must be protected from knocks and any other hazards on his transfer journey.

5 The nurse must accompany the patient and observe him closely for any changes in colour, breathing, and pulse-rate.

6 The wound dressing is checked for any soakage or staining.

Certain skills are acquired by the nurse so that she is able to deal with most emergencies as they occur.

The most important thing as that she should maintain the airway correctly.

This is minimised if the patient is on his side.

The nurse will be taught to elevate the chin so that it points forwards and upwards. In this way the tongue is not allowed to slip back.

An airway will normally be in position until the swallowing and coughing reflexes have recovered.

If vomiting occurs it is essential that the vomitus will not be inhaled. The top of the trolley for the transport of the patient must be able to be lowered for just such an emergency.

This is a very important part of the patient's care. The nurse must not neglect her duty in any way.

If she is in doubt about the Patient's condition she must summon help immediately.

Index

NOTES

NOTES

NOTES

NOTES

NOTES

NOTES

NOTES

NOTES

NOTES

NOTES

NOTES